Introduction

I've been using Bowen now since 2013 with great success with my clients. Since 2015 then I started to teach the Bowsage Method to massage therapists all over the country. My mentor, Dr. Mitchell Mosher, has graciously shared his many years of experience with me to continue to share with you how Bowen Techniques can positively impact you and your clients with a variety of physical, emotional and mental issues.

This course is a continuation of the Basic Bowen Technique exploring new Bowen techniques for specific illnesses, diseases and injuries. He has shared his experience with his own clients and how it helped them overcome and experience relief.

In this course we will also cover specifics in relation to the meridian system as it relates to the Chinese form of acupuncture and how those energy centers positively impact health issues. Learning about the meridian system and energy flow will help you, as a professional, understand how Bowen procedures open those lines of energy.

I hope you enjoy learning more about the powerful healing system of Bowen.

Table of contents:

- **Note from Michelle Lally**
- **About Dr. Mitchell Mosher**
- **About Thomas Bowen**
- **General Overview of Bowen**
    - Fascia system
    - Meridian Systems
    - Micro-Currents: The Direct Current System
    - Organ systems of Chinese Medicine
- **Basic Bowen Routine**
- **Advanced Bowen Procedures**
    - Arm Procedure 1
    - Arm Procedure 2
    - Shoulder
    - Cervical Release
    - Chairside Reboot
    - Deep Relaxation
    - Coccyx
    - Diaphragm
    - Digestive
    - Torso
    - Emotional Clearing
    - Hammertoes
    - Anterior Tibial Shin
    - Long Extensors
    - Peroneals
    - Bunion
    - Headache
    - Neck
    - Posterior Pelvis
    - Posterior Tibial
    - Sacral/Pregnant
    - Sciatica 1
    - Sciatica 2
    - Substance Dysfunction

- **CASE STUDIES:**
  - Allergies & Cravings
  - Ankle
  - Arthritis
  - Back Pain: Lower, Upper
  - Bedwetting
  - Bunions
  - Carpal Tunnel
  - Circulation
  - Colds & Flu, Sore throat
  - Colic
  - Coccyx
  - Depression
  - Digestive
  - Fibromyalgia
  - Heel Pain/Plantar Fasciitis
  - Infertility
  - Migraine
  - Neck pain
  - Parkinson's
  - Sciatica
  - Shoulder
  - Sinuses
  - TMJ
  - Tennis Elbow
  - Trauma
- Milton Albrecht Connection & the Bowen Technique

Note from Michelle Lally:
My teacher and lineage of Bowen Therapy comes from Dr. Mitchell Mosher who studied with Milton Albrecht who studied the Bowen Technique directly from Tom Bowen, the developer of Bowen Technique in Australia.

About Thomas Bowen:
Thomas Ambrose Bowen (1916-1982) began developing his technique in the 1950s in Geelong, Australia. He became interested in ways to alleviate human suffering and began to notice that certain moves on the body had particular effects. Tom Bowen developed his technique without having previous formal training in any modality or discipline. In fact, he frequently stated that his work was 'a gift from God'. He continued to develop and refine the technique throughout his lifetime with the help of his friend and secretary, Rene Horwood.

Mr. Bowen was extremely busy in his Geelong clinic, performing about 13,000 treatments a year. This was verified by the 1975 Victorian govern-ment inquiry into alternative health care professionals. Considering treatments were seven days apart and most people needed only one to three treatments, an amazing number of clients passed through the clinic and benefited from his gift. Mr. Bowen also held free clinics for children, people with disabilities, and community service workers.

In 1974, while attending a national health conference In Adelaide, Australia, Oswald Rentsch met Mr. Bowen for the first time. Although he knew nothing of Mr. Bowen's work, Ossie spontaneously asked if he could learn from him. Mr. Bowen shook Ossie's hand, held it for some time, and said, Good! Come down and I'll teach you.

In 1976, Ossie and his wife, Elaine, began utilizing Mr. Bowen's methods in their clinic in Hamilton, Victoria. Honoring Mr. Bowen's request to teach the work after his death, Ossie and Elaine named it the Bowen Technique and held their first seminar In Perth, Australia in 1986. By1990. Ossie and Elaine were teaching full time throughout Australia. Dedicated to preserving the technique and ensuring it was taught in its original form, they founded the Bowen Therapy Academy of Australia in 1987, eventually naming the technique Bowtech-The Bowen Technique.

Because this technique is so effective, it has been widely embraced internationally.

About Mitchell R. Mosher, DPM, LMBT
Health Consultant - Medical Bodywork - Retired Podiatrist
Roseville Podiatry From 1971 - 2006 · 35 years
Graduated California College of Podiatric Medicine
Teaching @ Family Practice Residents - UC Davis, CA
Author of: STRAYING FROM THE MAINSTREAM, A Doctor's Discoveries, & Bowen Therapy - Complete Practitioner's Guide

Mitchell practiced Podiatric Medicine & Foot Surgery. In 1995, he enhanced his practice by adding Bowen's Medical Bodywork, which added a whole new dimension to his life as well as his patient's.

From Dr. Moser's website: After serving in the army, I attended Marin Junior College prior to discovering my passion for helping alleviate people's pain and suffering through podiatry. I graduated Cum Laud from California College of Podiatric Medicine. I then completed a 2-year rotating medical internship and residency in foot surgery.

My residency included foot surgery, internal medicine, general and vascular surgery, pathology, anesthesiology, radiology, dermatology, and my favorite - Emergency & Trauma.

Because of this rich medical background, it enabled me to experiment with some Natural Health Options (Alternative Medicine) in my personal life and my podiatry practice, which is what led me to Tom Bowen's Bowen Technique.

After 12 years of trying absolutely everything short of surgery for severe back pain and spasms, one of my patients recommended a see a healer who was using a new technique (new to America), called Bowen Therapy. His name is Milton Albrecht who learned this technique directly from Tom Bowen. Needless to say, the rest is history as my pain eased, then disappeared. Of course, I had to learn this "magicical" healing system. And now, it is being passed down to you.

Mitchell R. Mosher, DPM, LMBT
Health Consultant - Medical Bodywork - Retired Podiatrist
Phone: 704-778-1740
Email: BowenFootDoc@gmail.com
Website: Bowen4Life.com

GENERAL OVERVIEW OF BOWEN THERAPY – by Dr. Mitchell Mosher

Bowen therapy is performed with loose fitting clothing, or if combining with a massage, you may use the sheets to affect the movements. It is best done with the client in a prone position followed by supine position, although it can be done sitting or standing as well based on the situation.

A series of "moves" are made over the fascia, muscles, tendons, and ligaments in specific locations with the fingers, thumbs, elbow, or side of the hand. The moves are made in a specific order, in designated places, and in a specific direction to obtain maximum results. The moves are very much like plucking a guitar string. Once plucked, the muscles and tendons vibrate from one end to the other, and from outside to inside. Subsequently, the muscle/tendon releases its holding pattern. Holding patterns occur to protect us from further injury. If you have ever experienced a whip-lash injury, chances are, when you look in the rear-view mirror and see a car coming upon your rear end while stopped at a stop light, you will instinctively tighten you neck to brace yourself from another injury. We remain on guard to protect against further traumas, which in turn is detrimental to our health.

Many of the moves are made over many "extraordinary" and "main meridian points", and along the meridian pathways. A series of moves makes up a procedure. Most procedures include a "Part A" and a "Part B". There are "rest periods" in between certain movements. These rests allow for the release of the primarily tightened muscles, the compensated muscles, the fascia, and the energy released from the entrapped compartments. Since many of the "moves" are along the meridian pathways, obstructions which were removed by the "moves" allow for the free flow of Qi energy, or Life Force. The rest periods give your body and energetic system time to take in the new data and processes it. After it has a chance to accept this information, it is then ready for additional data. At this point you may proceed with the next series of movements. Our cells are like silicon computer chips. They take in data and send out information. The rest periods during Bowen Therapy give the cells a chance to process the gentle stimuli and respond accordingly.

The basic relaxation procedures are located in the lower back, the upper back, shoulders and the neck. These movements over the nodal points release endorphins. For example, many of my patients tell me they can feel a "Runner's high, lightheadedness or euphoria after the treatment. Endorphins, discovered by a researcher, Candace Pert, PhD., are found to be the connecting link between the immune, endocrine, and central nervous systems. Tom Bowen concluded that 80% of the people, 80% of the time, would improve with these 3 simple procedures: Lower back, upper back/shoulders and neck. It is imperative to perform those first 3 procedures prior to any other series of movements. Once, I preformed Bowen on a client who was an acupuncturist. Afterwards, he said, "That's the closest thing to acupuncture that I've ever experienced, only without the needles!"

There are four reasons why I do an extensive Bowen Therapy session most of the time.

1. When I began my Bowen journey, I was only licensed to treat the muscles of the leg that affect the function of the feet. So, I did most of my sessions using the Lower Back BRM'S and the leg and foot procedures. These patients had good results for their foot, leg, knee, and hip problems.

    On occasion, patients would beg me to do their back, shoulders, and neck. Since I needed the practice and they needed the work, I would swear them to secrecy and go ahead and do a full sequence like what my teachers followed. That was from TMJ to Ankles and parts in between. Often, these patients had life changing events happen after their session. Also, their feedback on follow-up visits was much more positive than those who I did a limited session for.

    Over the years, I sometimes do upper back, neck and shoulder for shoulder problems. Or, upper back, neck, upper respiratory aka allergy/hay fever, and TMJ for jaw problems. These patients have good results for those problems too. But I can't recall a one of them who had a life changing experience like the many hundreds of patients had that I did a full sequence on.

2. The TMJ – Pelvis – Ankles are the main transverse plane (horizontal) balance points. If they are tilted or twisted, the alignment of all the frontal and sagittal plane structures become misaligned.

3. I believe that improving the function of the micro-current system – the 3rd dimension of the nervous system helps heal many old wounds and present issues. The micro-current system is a result of the cell membrane, fascia, and meridians.

    a. When fascia integrity is improved its liquid-crystal function is improved, hence more micro-currents generated and conducted.
    b. When fascia is loosened, the flow of micro-currents and bio chemicals along the meridian ductules are enhanced.

4. When bio-chemicals are released from the meridian points overall physiological function improves. For example; when clients tell us about the runner's high following a Bowen session, that's from the release of Beta Endorphins from the nodal points especially along the spine. Endorphins improve the communication links between the central, endocrine, and immune systems. For example; those clients who had a runner's high after their session, now report a new sense of peace, well-being, and balance.

FASCIAL SYSTEM

Fascia is a loose connective tissue compared with bone which is dense connective tissue. Besides a chain of connections between the skeletal parts of the musculoskeletal system, there is an even larger network of connective tissue which is interconnected amongst it called the fascial system. This system covers all structures, organs, and cells from head to toe, front to back, side to side and inside to outside. Think about piling thousands of full-body thermal suits on top of one another and connecting them together. That's about how the fascia system is. There is a superficial fascia from the base of the skull to the tips of the fingers and toes. Fat is attached to the outer layer, [panniculus adiposus] which is adjacent to an inner elastic layer both of which make up the superficial fascia. There is fascial surrounding the muscle compartments, muscle fascicles, muscle fibers, and myofibrils collectively called the myofascial, [Perimysium, Epimysium, Endomysium]. It has been estimated that the average human body contains approximately 65,000 linear miles of striated muscle fibers. Each fiber contains hundreds to thousands of myofibrils and myofilaments. Take an average of 1,000 and multiply X 65,000 = 65 million miles of myofascial in our bodies. Fascia surrounds the brain, the brainstem, and spinal cord called the Dural fascia. As the spinal nerves pass through the vertebral foramen the Dural fascia is re-named the myelin sheath of nerve. The lungs are coated with pleural fascia, the heart with pericardial fascia, the abdominal organs peritoneal fascia, the uro-genital organs with perineal fascia, the bone with periosteal fascia. Then, there are transverse bands of fascia from front to back and side to side; 1. In the floor of the pelvis, 2. The respiratory diaphragm, 3. Under the collarbone- the thoracic inlet, 4. Under the chin with hyoid fascia, 5. At the base of the cranium with cranial base fascia, and 6. Joint capsules. In addition, there is a thin veil of fascia adjacent to the cytoskeleton of every non-circulating cell in the body as well as para tendons, and retinaculum's. That's a whole lot of tissue all connected to one another. These connective tissues allow the body to maintain shape, protect the structures from outside forces, and some scholars feel it aids in cellular functions such as respiration, digestion, reproduction, and excretion. I believe that the fascia is a component of the 3rd dimension of the nervous system which is described in the section on the direct currents.

HISTOLOGY & PHYSIOLOGY OF FASCIA

The fascia is made up of 3 significant structures. Collagen, elastin, and a ground substance consisting of a colloid gel matrix which contains hyaluronic acid and mucopolysaccharides. The collagen part provides the protective-supportive function. The colloid gel acts as a shock absorber. And, the elastin allows for stretch. There are 2 other properties of the fascia which are of vital importance, neither of which are discussed in medical physiology books at my last search. First, the collagen has 3 protein strands, one of which is a crystalline band. All crystalline structures can generate piezoelectricity. "Piezo" means push in Greek. When the fascia is stretched direct currents [positive cations] are pushed out of the crystalline strand, and when the fascia is compressed [negative anions] are pushed out of the crystalline strands. Secondly, the colloid gel is thixotropic. This means that the gel can convert to a liquid when heated or stretched, and then returns to a gel when cooled. Combined together, we have within us a liquid, [conductor] - crystal, [generator] system, which can generate and conduct D.C.'s, [direct currents].

Orthodontia is based on this piezoelectric effect. When the bands are applied and stress is transmitted through the tooth down into the boney socket, piezoelectricity is generated from 2 structures. One, is the periosteum [connective tissue/fascia], which has a crystalline strand in the protein part of the collagen. The second, is the hydroxy appetite crystalline part of the bone [connective tissue]. Dr. Becker applied stress to dead bones and found that they were capable of generating direct currents. Thus, the production of positive and negative micro-current charges stimulate the cellular activities which are instrumental in the remodeling of the bone.

FASCIAL UNWINDING

In the myofascial system, which comes first? The Myo, or the fascia? During my surgical career, when dissecting the fascia, it was virtually impossible to separate the muscle tissue from the fascial tissue without sacrificing a little of one or the other. It matters not which is which, but that they both unwind as a result of the Reflex Arcs. I witness this frequently on the Rhomboid Muscles after the "Boomerang Moves" in the upper back procedure. While doing the first moves, nodules can often be palpated. When the moves are repeated a few minutes later, the nodules are usually gone completely, or at least significantly reduced.

I have also witnessed the unwinding to continue for many years after the patient's last session. I believe that two important things occur during and after the unwinding; 1. the muscles elongate and develop improved function, 2. the fascia becomes anatomically aligned. Multiple other changes follow these first two; A. there can be a release of lactic acid build up, B. the meridians that pass through the fascia can flow more freely, C. emotional memories can be released from the fascia, D. piezoelectric and thixotropic function is restored, and, E. entrapped energies [energy cysts] are freed. The following two case histories will demonstrate these phenomenon:

One of my more interesting experiences occurred with a patient and his responses, which took place the very first week I started doing Bowen. Another Podiatrist down the road who was not able to help him referred Bernard to me. Bernard had an arthritic large toe joint, which he did not want to have surgery on. He told me that he was favoring the toe and this was making his hip and back painful. He was hopeful that some type of shoe modification would suffice to relieve his problems. His joint was red, swollen, tender, and with movement grated like sand paper [crepitus]. I informed him that I could accommodate his shoe and for him to leave it over the weekend and I would get it done. Then I told him about the Bowen treatment, which might relieve the pains in his hip and back. He begged me to also perform the upper back and neck moves and promised he would not tell anyone [that was before I obtained a massage certificate- and my podiatry license only covered the leg muscles]. I felt comfortable with him, so I did a complete treatment from head to toe. When I had finished the procedures, I had learned in class, I examined his Extensor Hallucis Longus Muscles. The one on the right side was like a rope. So, I figured that if they had taught a procedure on this in class, it would be slack to the table and make an anterior move, good side first. So, I did the left side 1st, and then did the right-side muscle, and he immediately let out a moan. I asked if he was all right, and he said, "I am alright. It kind of hurt and tickled at the same time". I left the room for a few minutes in order to let him rest and for the release to take place. When I returned, he was curled up in a fetal position and was quite pale and cold. My first thought was that he had fainted and was going into shock. I checked his pulse and was going to take his blood pressure when he said," I'm okay. I'm a little cold. May I have a blanket"? I covered him up and left him alone to settle down for a few minutes. When I returned his color was a little better, but he was still chilled. I left him to lie on the table for a few more minutes. The next time I returned to check on him he was sitting on the edge of the table looking a little haggard, but much better. I gave him his post-treatment instructions and told him to pick up his shoe on Monday. When I saw him in the waiting room Monday morning prior to appointment times I said, "Hi Bernard. I've got your shoe ready". He said very emphatically, "I don't care about the shoe. I want to know when I can get another treatment." I said, "That's right I gave you a Bowen last week. How did it work?" He said, "How did it work? It changed my life. The past 3 nights have been the only full night's sleep I have had in years. My back does not hurt. The pain in my hip is all but gone and look at my toe"! He commenced to remove his shoe and sock and bend the toe up and down and said, "See. Look at this." I could not help but walk out into the waiting room and look at his toe up close. The swelling, redness and crepitus were completely resolved. There remained a little stiffness but the toe flexed at least 50% more than it did on Friday. I told him that he could make an appointment for Friday.

When he returned the following Friday, I asked how he was doing and he said, "I am doing fantastic. I don't have any more stress, I am more focused, and I feel like I've been liberated from something that had a hold of me". He went on to tell me that the day before he had given notice at the job he had loathed, and was moving to Costa Rica within the next month to open a restaurant. This was something that he had wanted to do for quite some time but something was holding him back. He said," Whatever you did that treatment last week released whatever it was that was holding me down". At the time, I was not quite sure what had just transpired because they did not teach us at the Bowen workshop I took, anything about this emotional release stuff. After a couple of more experiences, and conversations with other therapists I finally got a clue about it all. When I checked his right EHL Muscle, the rope was gone.

Another somatic emotional release experience was with a young lady who was referred to me by a foot surgeon a few miles away. He knew that I did Bowen Therapy, and his patient was suffering with chronic back pain. She had been examined and treated by competent doctors and nothing had relieved her pain. So, she wanted to try a Bowen treatment, which she had heard about since she was a Massage Therapist. Her first session was uneventful. She felt only minimal relief of the pain. She returned 2 weeks later for another session. I began with the basic relaxation moves, then did the kidney and lower respiratory moves. Then, when I returned to the room following the 4-minute rest after releasing the abdominal muscles, she was quietly weeping. I asked if she was all right and if she needed a blanket. She said that she was little cold and a blanket would be nice. I said, 'It looks like you are releasing something. Do you want to talk about it or keep it to yourself"? She said, I'll tell you what it is. I had a caesarian section 2 years ago and it was against my will. My mother and the doctors pretty much forced me to have it and I've been angry ever since. I felt like I was invaded by aliens". After the session she was completely pain free, relaxed and has been fine ever since. This illustrates how the abdominal area is the "Front of the Back". And, how the fascia is all interrelated.

We all need to keep in mind that all of the musculoskeletal structures, including the fascia and myofascial are all connected to one another. The position and motions taking place in the feet-affect the legs, hips, pelvis, back, shoulder, neck, and head. And, twists, tilts, angulations of the pelvis- affect the feet and ankles, as well as proximal structures. Therefore, when a practitioner stimulates a release in the front, that results in a change in the back. When a release takes place at the bottom, a change takes place at the top. Lastly, when there are releases to superficial structures, changes take place in the deeper parts. This also explains why the Coccyx locks and Kidney moves help digestive disorders in adults and colic in babies. I do these along with other abdominal and torso moves for patients undergoing chemotherapy. As long as I do them once a week, they have zero nausea symptoms. If we skip a week, they experience severe nausea, and can't wait for their next session.

MICRO-CURRENTS - THE DIRECT CURRENT SYSTEM

"The Other Nervous System" The 3rd Dimension

Our body electric is much like our homes. 110 Volt & 220 Volt systems operate many of our household appliances, computers, heaters, water pumps, lights and stereos. Direct Current (D.C.) with positive and negative polarities powers the smoke detectors, doorbells, intercoms, and stereo speakers. These electrical currents travel via wiring systems which are turned on and off with switches and breakers and are modulated by transformers, capacitors and resisters, and reducers.

Our body operates in a similar fashion. The 1st dimension is the central nervous system. The 2nd dimension is the peripheral nervous system consisting of the Voluntary nervous system (sensory and motor nerves) and the Involuntary/Autonomic nervous system (sympathetic and parasympathetic nerves), and my belief is that there is a 3rd dimension which is, the Direct Current (D.C.) system. The D.C system is probably conducted via the meridian ductile system, nerve sheath [myelin sheath], intra-cellular and extra-cellular water, and the colloid gel matrix of the fascia. Some data has been gathered by Dr. Robert O. Becker and Bruce Lipton, PhD, which supports this probability. The collagen within the fascia is made up from proteins which contains crystalline strands. These crystalline structures generate piezoelectricity. This is one of the systems that creates micro-currents. Another generator is the cell membrane system. The micro-currents are instrumental in modulating wound and tissue repair, healing of fractures, bone and scar remodeling, and cellular regeneration by way of influencing cellular activities. Our body electric has been measured and has shown a positive polarity through the central nervous system and the central part of the physical body. The extremities and peripheral tissues consist of negative polarity; an unfertile egg also is positive in the middle and negative on the perimeter. So are a hydrogen atom and a water molecule.

The effects of positive and negative polarity on cellular and tissue activities have been studied extensively around the world during the past 50 years, or more.

POSITIVE / CATIONS = MOSTLY ANTIBIOLOGICAL / CATABOLIC
1. Anticarcinogenic – reverses cancer
2. Attracts macrophages – cells that clean up debris / release endorphins
3. Bacteriostatic – stops reproduction of organisms
4. Bactericidal if combined with silver ions – kills organisms
5. Causes bone resorption (Wolf's Law of Bone)
6. Denatures protein
7. Prevents post ischemic lipid per oxidation
8. Promotes epithelial growth and organization
9. Reduces keloids and scars
10. Reduces fibrosis
11. Reduces tensile strength of wounds
12. Repels mast cells – inflammation and allergy cells
13. Retards biological growth
14. Stimulates osteoclastic activity- cells that resorb bone
15. Vasoconstrictive

NEGATIVE / ANIONS = MOSTLY BIOLOGICAL / ANABOLIC

1. Attracts neutrophils – cells that fight infection.
2. Decreases edema – swelling.
3. Increases fibroblastic activity - cells that form collagen.
4. Increases fibroblastic proliferation and collagen formation.
5. Increases growth factor receptor sites on fibroblasts.
6. Increases repair and regeneration.
7. Induces epidermal cell migration.
8. Lyses necrotic tissue – dead tissue.
9. Stimulates granulation tissue.
10. Stimulates osteocytes (bone marrow cells) to migrate to a fracture site in order to form crystalline hydroxy apatite for the formation of calcium for fracture repair or bone remodeling.
11. Stimulates osteoblastic activity-cells that form bone matrix.
12. Stimulates dendrite formation directionally.
13. Vasodilatation.

Dr. Robert O. Becker, M.D. found that when one cuts a finger, the negative polarity shifts to positive for about 5 days. Following that, the polarity shifts back to negative and increases in amperage until day 21, at which time the polarity gradually returns to its normal resting state. Wound repair takes place, generally as follows. At the time of the cut platelets clump, a band aid and compression is applied, and the cations constrict the capillaries all of which help to stop the bleeding. The cations also help to keep the wound from infection due to its bacteriostatic effects. A thrombin clot with aid of fibrinogen seals the wound and forms a scaffold for further healing by collagen. Cations stimulate macrophages which clean up the dead cells and debris at the wound site. All of this transpires during the first 5 days. Next, negative anion microcurrents intensify during the next 14 to 16 days and attract the fibroblasts to come to the wound site, proliferate, open receptor sites for hormone peptide growth factors, and form pro-collagen and collagen (super-glue) as a result of the anions. Usually at about day 21 the wound has its maximum tensile strength so the anions lower back down to the normal basal resting state. That's why there is pruritis, [itching] at the wound or injury site from around day 14 to day 21. Then, for the next 6 months to 1 year the scar re-organizes. If you check the effects of the currents, they pretty much correlate to the phases of wound repair. I speculate that if Dr. Becker had carried on his measurements at the wound site for months after, he probably would have charted intense positive charges which are responsible for the resorption of scar tissue.

Doctor Becker wanted to know what structures or circuits these currents flowed through and performed the following experiment. He removed a section of the sciatic nerve from the leg in a rat and then confirmed the de-nerving by nerve conduction studies to the distal fibula. He then fractured the distal fibula [outer ankle bone]. He noted that even though the nerve had not reconnected by the time the fractures had healed, the fracture healed in spite. Although the fracture healing time was delayed 2 to 4 weeks. He then studied 3 groups of rats, where the 1st group he sectioned the nerve and waited 5 days to fracture the bone, the 2nd group he waited 10 days, and the 3rd group he waited 15 days. All 3 groups healed in the usual 4 weeks time. He concluded that something happened the 1st five days. He then severed the nerve in another rat, waited 5 days, and then took the wound apart. He visualized a thin film of tissue bridging the gap between the cut nerve ends. When he looked at the tissue with a microscope he observed Schwann cells, which are the main cells of the nerve sheath myelin sheath]. Therefore, the nerve sheath probably conducts the D.C. flow or, possibly the meridian that runs along the nerve as we will discover later. Or, possibly the fascia is the conductor, as the fascia surrounds every cell in the body, and the nerve sheath is really a brand of connective fascial tissue.

Doctor Becker made an interesting observation. Over all of the years that he performed experiments on animals, fracturing bones and observing them heal; they never had a non-union of a fracture. He did not immobilize the limbs either. No casts, no pins, plates, or screws. He let them run around the cages and there were only mal-unions and delayed unions. He said, "Only people get non-unions". About 1:1,000, even though they are immobilized internally, and or externally. He did not pursue this notion, but I have pondered it and my theory is that animals; have less stress, follow a natural diet, and do a lot of stretching. The stretching maintains fascial integrity and resultant piezoelectricity & thixotropy. How many times a day do you see the average person stretch? How many times a day do you stretch? Animals stretch every chance they get.

MERIDIANS

The meridians are; .5 to 1.5 micron (1/1,000 mm.) in diameter ducts which carry bioenergy; Qi - pronounced "Chee" in China, Ki - pronounced "Key" in Japan and Korea, Pranna - pronounced "Prah Na" in the Mid East, and Life Force - in North America.

Qi consists of electrical currents, probably direct current, D.C., chemicals, and maybe more. There are 14 main meridians, 12 of which have peak cycles during 2 hour time spans during the course of the day. The meridians cycle as follows;

Liver 1:00 A.M. to 3:00 A.M.

Lung 3:00 A.M. to 5:00 A.M.

Large Intestine 5:00 A.M. to 7:00 A.M.

Stomach 7:00 A.M. to 9:00 A.M.

Spleen 9:00 A.M. to 11:00 A.M.

Heart 11:00 A.M. to 1:00 P.M.

Small Intestine 1:00 P.M. to 3:00 P.M.

Urinary Bladder 3:00 P.M. to 5:00 P.M.

Kidney 5:00 P.M. to 7:00 P.M.

Pericardium 7:00 P.M. to 9:00 P.M.

Triple warmer 9:00 P.M. to 11:00 P.M.

Gallbladder 11:00 PM to 1:00 A.M.

The other 2 main meridians are the conception vessel in the front of the body and the governing vessel in the back. These meridians cycle continuously around the clock. There are numerous other collateral and distribution meridians throughout the body.

The meridians are anatomically laid out like our freeway, hi-way, by-way, street, alleyway, cull de sac systems. The meridians function like an irrigation canal system, a very slow flowing non-pressurized system. They've been measured to flow at a rate of approximately 12 inches in 4 to 8 minutes depending on which meridian is measured. This is very slow compared to the blood circulatory system, which circulates from ventricle to atrium in 14 seconds, in a normal person at rest. The meridians have been observed in chick embryos, with the aid of high-resolution microscopy and a gamma ray scanner following injection of a radioisotope. The entire system is laid out and is fully developed within 15 hours following conception. Dr. Gerber cites studies that suggest that the etheric energy field directs the formation of the meridian system. And, that the development of the body parts and organ arrangement is determined by the meridians. Otherwise, how would the heart know to develop here and the liver over there? These channels appear before any vessels, nerves, organs, or limb buds.

In another study performed in Korea, the researcher removed a portion of the liver meridian and followed up with fine needle biopsies of the liver tissues. He noted the beginning of degeneration of hepatocytes (liver cells), after 3 days. Therefore, the meridians are crucial for development and regeneration and repair.

The meridians have been isolated by a French researcher who injected a radioisotope (technetium 99) into humans at the meridian points and at random meridian points in the skin. He observed the ductile systems with a microscope connected to a gamma ray camera and notes that there is a superficial system under the skin and 4 deep systems; (1.along the vessels and lymph channels, 2. along the nerves, 3. inside the blood vessels, and 4.through the spaces around the internal organs) all of which are interconnected with each other and the superficial system by way of collaterals.

The meridian points have been biopsied by several researchers and the following is a summary of their findings:
1. The points are adjacent to a corpuscle *diaphragm*.
2. Beneath the corpuscle is a plexus of nerves and blood vessels.
3. Biochemical analysis of tissue fluids reveal:

>10 times the amount of adrenalin than is in the blood.
>Amino acids.
>Cortisone.
>DNA & RNA.
>Hyaluronic acid.
>16 different free nucleotides.
>estrogens, endorphins, and kinins.

Additionally, Dr. Becker studied the meridians with respect to their electrical activity. There is a measurable direct current flowing throughout, at some points positive and others negative. The amperage dropped as the probe was moved along the meridian pathway and when the probe reached a meridian point the amperage increased. It is thought that the points are like transformers, which boost the flow of the currents, because electrical current loses velocity as it travels distance.

As the meridians and nerves pass through the fascial structures and while the fascial-periosteal structures conduct the liquid-crystal system, it doesn't take a rocket scientist to figure out that prolonged fascial / myofascial dysfunction may cause occlusions in the direct current bioelectrical system. Prolonged bioelectrical dysfunction will lead to cellular and biochemical dysfunction. Prolonged cellular and biochemical dysfunction may cause signs, symptoms, deformities, and disabilities. Additionally, fascial / myofascial dysfunction can lead to neuromuscular pain and skeletal misalignments. Therefore, removal of myofascial and fascial dysfunctions will improve the bioelectrical / biochemical functions which in turn will affect the cellular and biochemical functions, in addition to relieving neuromuscular pain, and deforming forces on the tissues. The reflex arcs from Bowen moves probably do all of this.

It makes you wonder how the Easterners knew all about the systems without any high- tech. They appeared to have mapped out the meridian and meridian point system about 4,000 years ago. However, when the frozen Eastern European hunter named "Itzy" sic, (discovered in a thawing glacier in Easter Europe), was carbon dated it was found that he was 5,500 years old. He had rheumatoid arthritis of the spine when they did the autopsy. Rheumatologists became very excited to learn that rheumatoid arthritis was not a modern age illness. They also found tattoos on his body placed over the meridian points which you would treat for pain in the areas where he had the arthritic processes. So, this was known about approximately 1,500 years before Qi Boy convinced the emperor of the Yellow Dynasty that acupuncture should be added to the Chinese Medicine formulary! A case that will reveal the re-establishment of meridian flow and subsequent healing of a chronic problem follows:

One Monday morning, a few months following my first Bowen class, a patient presented with a lump the size of an almond beneath the arch on the right foot. She told me that there was very little pain involved however, she was favoring it and this was causing pains in her hip and lower back. She was also concerned because we are all suspicious when a "lump" appears. I reassured her that the lump was a classical benign plantar fibroma. Only if it grew rapidly or became painful should she consider having it removed. I informed her about the therapy that I had recently discovered and that it could help her back and hip. She immediately took me up on my offer. When we were all finished, she arose from the table and said, "Oh my, I feel so good. Can I come back tomorrow for another treatment?" I told her that we should wait one week before another session and for her to make an appointment.

When she returned the following week, the lump had reduced to the size of a pea and she said that she couldn't wait for another Bowen treatment. She scheduled another check on her foot and Bowen session one week later.

I began the therapy prior to looking at her foot. During a point where the muscles are released on the inner thigh area she asked, "Is there any connection between that lump on my foot and my stomach?" I said, "I don't think so. Why?" She replied, "On the first visit when you released those muscles in the inner part of my thigh and left the room for me to rest, I immediately felt like a gush of worms crawling around in my stomach. All day long, I had a queasy feeling in my stomach. In addition, when I got home from work that night my stomach and gallbladder pain completely disappeared. I've not had to take any of my stomach medications for the past three weeks. I flushed $200 worth of prescriptions down the toilet this morning. When I get to work, I'm calling the gastroenterologist who has been taking care of me the past two years and canceling my appointment for the endoscope procedure at the surgery center next week." She had an endoscopy procedure done every six months to keep a check on her problem! She added, "I won't need him any more." I begged her not to mention my connection with any of this, as I didn't want to be in any trouble with the medical community or lose any referrals due to my deviating from the main stream. She assured me that she wouldn't and then she said, "Look at my foot." As I looked for the lump, it was almost completely gone. Now, it was about the size of a grain of rice! I found an old foot reflexology book and opened to the foot chart. Sure enough, the lump was right in the middle of the stomach and liver zone. I told her about that and she laughed, left the office quite happy, and has never returned.

Two years later, I was studying Acupuncture and recalled the incident. When I looked at the meridian chart, I saw that two of the four meridians that pass through the inner thigh and groin are the Stomach and Liver meridians. I could chalk it all up to coincidence or spontaneous remission. Or, I could believe that there was some kind of obstruction in that muscle tissue of the adductor canal and inguinal ligament which was blocking the flow of energy. When the blockage was released due to the immediate unwinding as a result of the reflex arcs, she then felt the "Gush of worms into her stomach". Then, she healed herself. I tend to believe in the later. What is most perplexing is that the pathology reports following biopsy of these fibrous lesions in the plantar foot area always state, "Benign fibroplasia. Multiple fibroblasts and swirls of collagen." I'm not sure as to how this scar-like tissue could recede in three weeks. But, it did.

Organ Systems of Chinese Medicine

Zang – Fu Organs in Traditional Chinese Medicine

The concept of the organs in Traditional Chinese Medicine (TCM) is radically different from that of contemporary western medicine. Understanding this difference is very important because the physiology and pathology of the Organs is fundamental to the understanding and treatment of disease. Chinese medical theory is not a quick study, but we have tried to break it down for you throughout this website so that you can be a better advocate for your own health and well-being. For best outcomes using self-care, combine associated Aroma Acu-Sticks® to acu-points, organic herbs, topical remedies, and good lifestyle practices.

Zang – The Yin organs Kidney, Liver, Heart (Pericardium), Spleen, and Lungs are considered as deeper than the Yang organs, generally more solid, and are involved with the regulation, manufacturing and storage of fundamental substances such as Blood and Essence.

Fu – The Yang organs Stomach, Gall Bladder, Large Intestine, Small Intestines, Bladder, and San Jiao are the hollow organs are viewed as being closer to the surface, or exterior of the body. They are not store substances, and are instead involved with an ongoing process of change through functions of receiving, separating, distributing, and excreting substances.

Kidney Organ System of Chinese Medicine

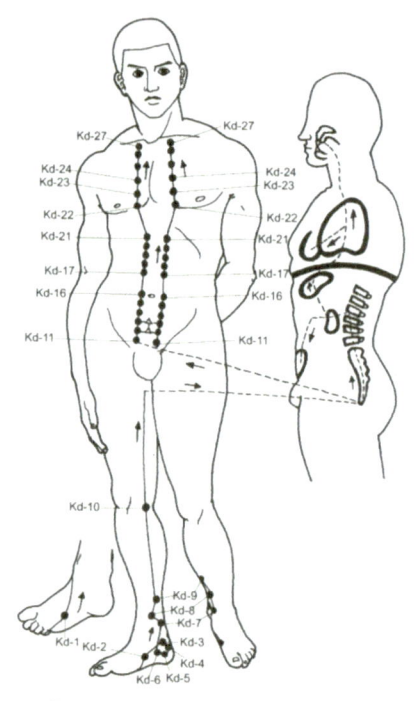

- Controls the waterways and regulates fluid balance in the body.
- Stores the Essences (Jing) and produces marrow; this 'Bone Marrow' is essential in the formation of bone, the spinal cord, Blood, and the brain.
- Is the base of all Yin and Yang of the body and maintain the Gate of Vitality, or Mingmen Fire.
- Open into the ear and influence hearing, and manifest in the hair reflecting Kidney health through vital, lush, shiny hair.

Common Symptoms of Kidney Imbalances

- Afternoon and night sweats
- Low energy
- Fear, panic attacks, phobias and anxiety
- Premature aging including graying of hair
- Memory loss
- Sexual dysfunctions including impotence
- Infertility
- Urinary disorder

The Internal and External Qi Flow of the Kidney (Kd) Channels

Liver Organ System

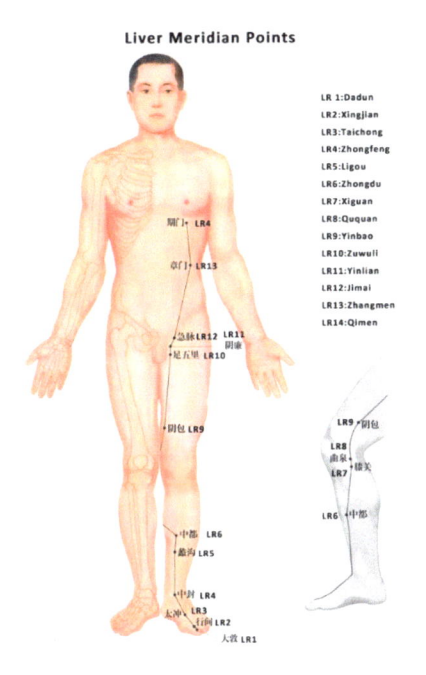

- Opens in to the eyes providing nourishing Liver Blood for vision health.
- Spread Qi of all organs in all directions and allows the free flow of Qi throughout the body necessary for the healthy function of the body.
- Stores Blood and regulates the amount of Blood in circulation, storing and releasing it as bodily demands present themselves.
- Controls tendons and nourishes the tendons and joints with Liver Blood.

Common Symptoms of Liver Imbalances
- Headaches, PMS, anger and frustration
- Acid reflux
- Irritable Bowel Syndrome (IBS)
- Osteo-arthritis and stiff joints
- Brittle nails
- Lack of vision and direction in planning one's life

Heart Organ System

- Governs all emotion
- Sexual warmth
- Controls blood vessels

Common Symptoms of Heart Imbalances
- Emotional instability
- Insomnia
- Palpitations
- Heart disease
- Poor memory
- Mouth and tongue ulcers

Spleen Organ System

- Controls the raising of Qi
- Contains the Blood
- Transforms and transports foods and fluids

Common Symptoms of Spleen Imbalances
- Poor appetite
- Gas and abdominal distension
- Dampness
- Tiredness or weakness
- Loose stools
- Prolapsed organs
- Uterine bleeding
- Varicose veins
- Easy bruising
- Obsessive worry
- Lack of empathy

Lung Organ System

- Receives the Qi from the heavens
- Governs over the skin and hair
- Open into the nose
- Controls immune system

Common Symptoms of Lung Imbalances
- Coughing
- Bronchitis, asthma
- COPD
- Sinusitis
- Frequent colds or flu
- Sadness or unresolved grief
- Dogmatism
- Lack of self-worth
- Poor personal boundaries

Chinese Medical Concept of Energetic Organ Systems

To a modern westerner, the Chinese concept of organs might seem unusual as the Chinese medical concept of organs lack emphasis on a physical structure. Although many terms used when speaking of organs are similar to western concepts, they do not always refer to the specific organ tissue or structure, but rather to semi-abstract concepts of interrelated functions.
Each organ system has an impact on the other organ systems when it becomes imbalanced; additionally, each organ has an impact on the emotions. Chinese medicine views the individual person as a whole, interactive entity rather than individual parts and pieces. This is how Chinese medicine is able to differentiate disease patterns and devise effective treatment strategies. One disease can have many different patterns depending on a person's individual body make-up, genetic dispositions, and lifestyle habits. The functions listed are not based on surgical discoveries, but on clinical observation of patients over many thousands of years, making Chinese medicine very practical in actual application.

References https://agelessherbs.com/organ-systems-of-chinese-medicine/

LIVE AS IF!

What is the one thing I could teach another massage therapist that could improve their practice?
The answer is simple "Live as if."
What does "Live as if" stand for?
It means that we create the life, the business and the customers we dream of having. Live as if your goals are already met. Whether it means that you are the most compassionate massage therapist offering care to those who can't afford it, or most successful with other therapists working for you, or you're the most educated body-worker in your community. Whatever your personal and professional goals are, live as if they have already come true.
We hear people say "I don't have time to get a massage" or "I don't have time to take another class." Yet too often these are health industry professionals who want to attract the kind of person, client or patient that sees the value of self-care. Make a choice to be the person you want to attract to your life, personal or professional. Surround yourself with a community of people who do the same.
For example, I receive a weekly massage, from a therapist who also receives massage, or in other ways takes care of themselves. They believe as I do that it is the most important thing they can do, in addition to other self-care therapies and healthy living regimens. So, I attract customers who also believe in self-care practices.

Ten things to be mindful of
1. 10 swallows of water! Most people put a cup to the mouth and maybe swallow 3 or 4 times, stop and take 10 swallows (of water) each time you put a cup to your lips.
2. 10 Breaths ~breathe in and out ten times don't stop
3. 10 min Stretch as often as you can each day for at least
4. 10 min Meditation that's all it takes, think of something your grateful for, you can compassion for, you feel love for
5. 10 Affirmations~ just ask google/siri/alexa to tell you 10 if you can't think of any.
6. 10 min of walking ~in place counts too, make sure you swing your arms
7. 10 min of smiling ~at yourself in the mirror, your dog, a stranger whatever works…
8. 10 min of feet on the ground (no shoes)
9. 10 acts of kindness (that can mean throwing a love/peace hand sign instead of what you really wanted to
10. 10 min call a friend you have not spoken to, or relative

When I look back on my success as a Bowen Therapy Instructor, Massage Therapist and Retreat Owner, I can attribute it to learning one simple tool:
Live as if!
I have had my own Wellness Center, working with other healthy lifestyle professionals who believe as I do about quality of care for themselves, their family and their community. I attract clients who are seeking a healthy lifestyle and also give back to their community through donations, gift cards or reduced rates for the elderly.
My massage career started at 42, now I'm 60, have two adult children, grandchildren, a loving partner, perfect home/retreat, a successful business and I practice self-care daily. My key to a happy, healthy and abundant lifestyle?
I live as if!
Published in 2018 Massage Magazine

OTHER WAYS OF HELPING YOUR TRIBE/COMMUNITY

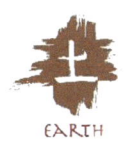

Earth - Spleen and Stomach Channel
Acupressure Points can affect- Spleen and Stomach Channel address digestive issues, Earth Element such as worry, overthinking, and lack of empathy. Ingredients Earth Coconut Oil, Juniper, Tangerine, Spearmint, Fennel and Ginger Essential Oils

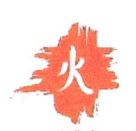

Fire - Heart-Pericardium Channel
Acupressure Points can affect. Fire Element of Chinese medicine such as lack of joy. emotional/sexual coldness, emotional/Shen disorders, and sleep problems. Ingredients Fire Coconut Oil, Lavender, Sweet Orange, Frankincense and Rose Essential Oils

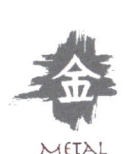

Metal Element- Lung-Large Intestine Channell
Acupressure Points can affect Many of the points along both Channels help to normalize the respiratory system including the sinuses. Addresses issues associated with Metal Element Imbalances including unresolved grief and sadness, lack of spiritual connection or growth, digestive issues, poor personal boundaries, and low self-worth. Ingredients Metal Coconut Oil, Bergamot, Sweet Orange, Oregano, Cypress and Cinnamon Essential Oils.

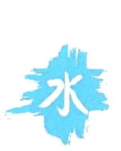

Water Element- Kidney-Bladder Channel
Acupressure Points can affect the Kidney and Bladder Meridians. Water Element of Chinese medicine such as lack of willpower, lack of awe, anxiety, and irrational fears leading to panic attacks. This blend activates acupressure points that assist with issues such as low virility and infertility as well as other Kidney energetic attributes such as premature aging. Ingredients Water Coconut Oil, Lavender, Cinnamon, Eucalyptus, Wintergreen, Sweet Orange, Helichrysum, Clove and Peppermint Essential Oils.

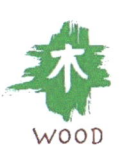

Wood Element - Liver-Gallbladder
Acupuncture acupressure points can affect the Liver and Gallbladder Meridians. Can alleviate emotional constraints leading to depression, anger and frustration as well as physical maladies associated with the Wood Element imbalances according to Chinese medicine such as menstrual disorders and poor sleep patterns. Wood Coconut Oil, Lavender, Rosemary, Cedarwood and Lemongrass Essential Oils.

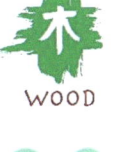

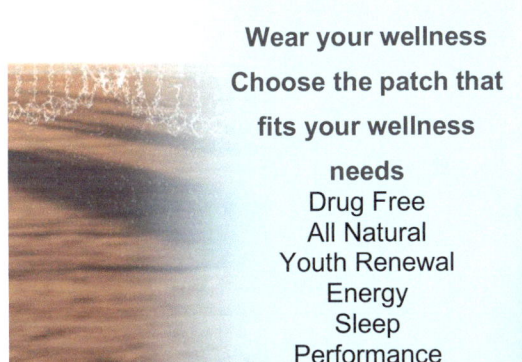

Wear your wellness
Choose the patch that
fits your wellness
needs
Drug Free
All Natural
Youth Renewal
Energy
Sleep
Performance
Fast Pain Relief

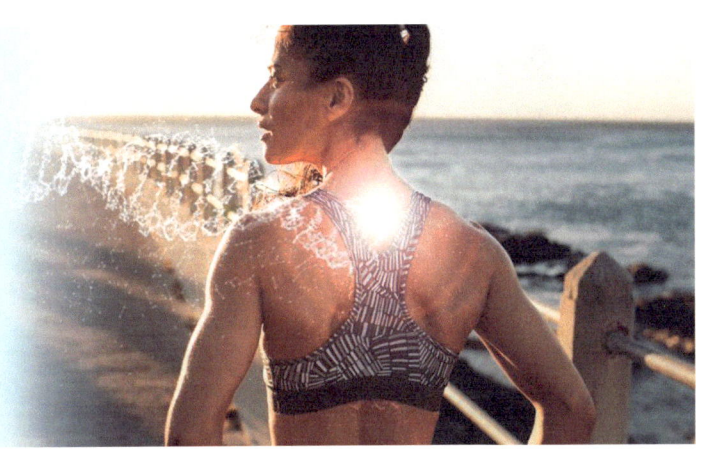

95% of the Bowen Moves are done over the Meridian System

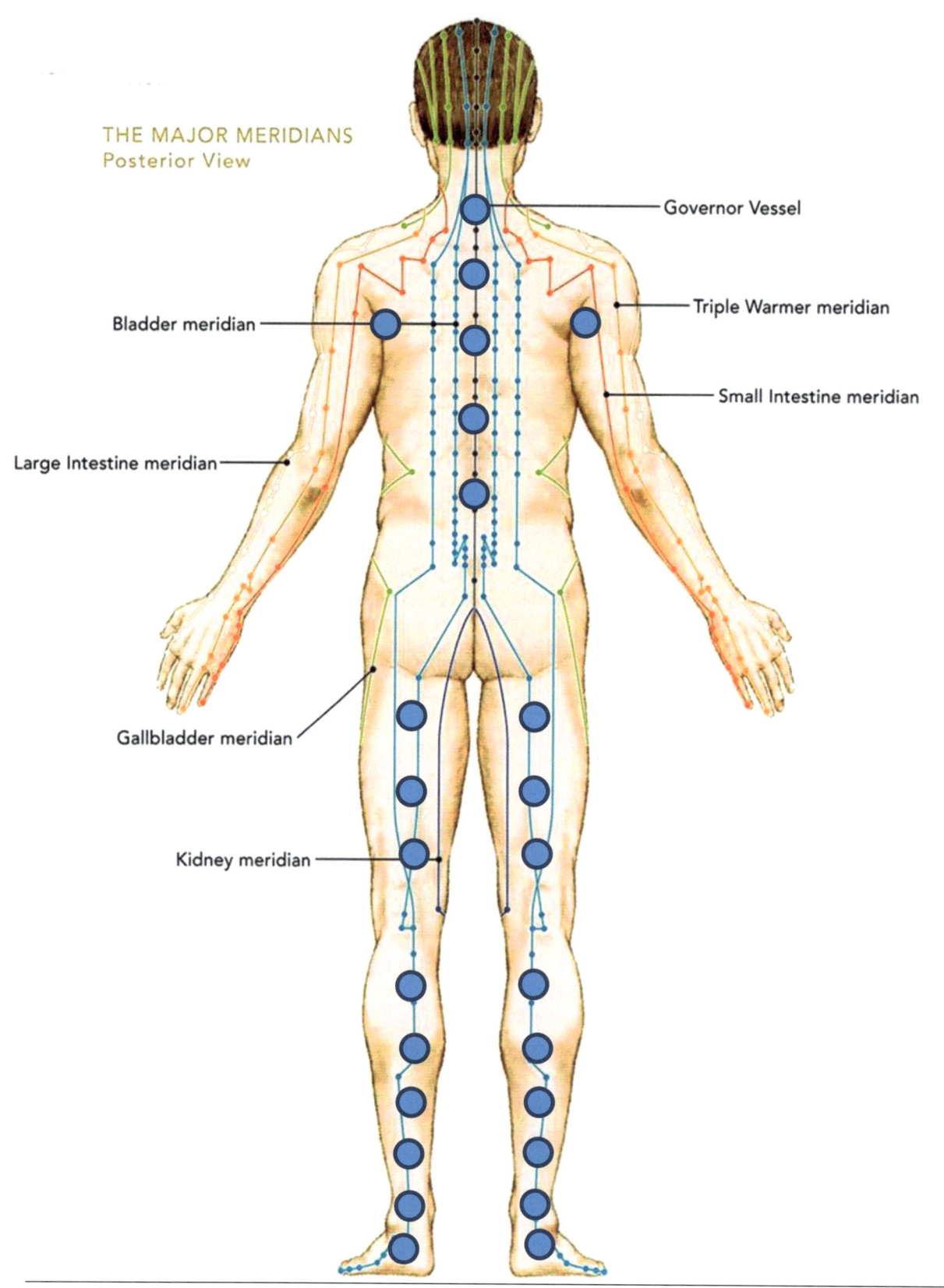

THE MAJOR MERIDIANS
Posterior View

- Governor Vessel
- Triple Warmer meridian
- Bladder meridian
- Small Intestine meridian
- Large Intestine meridian
- Gallbladder meridian
- Kidney meridian

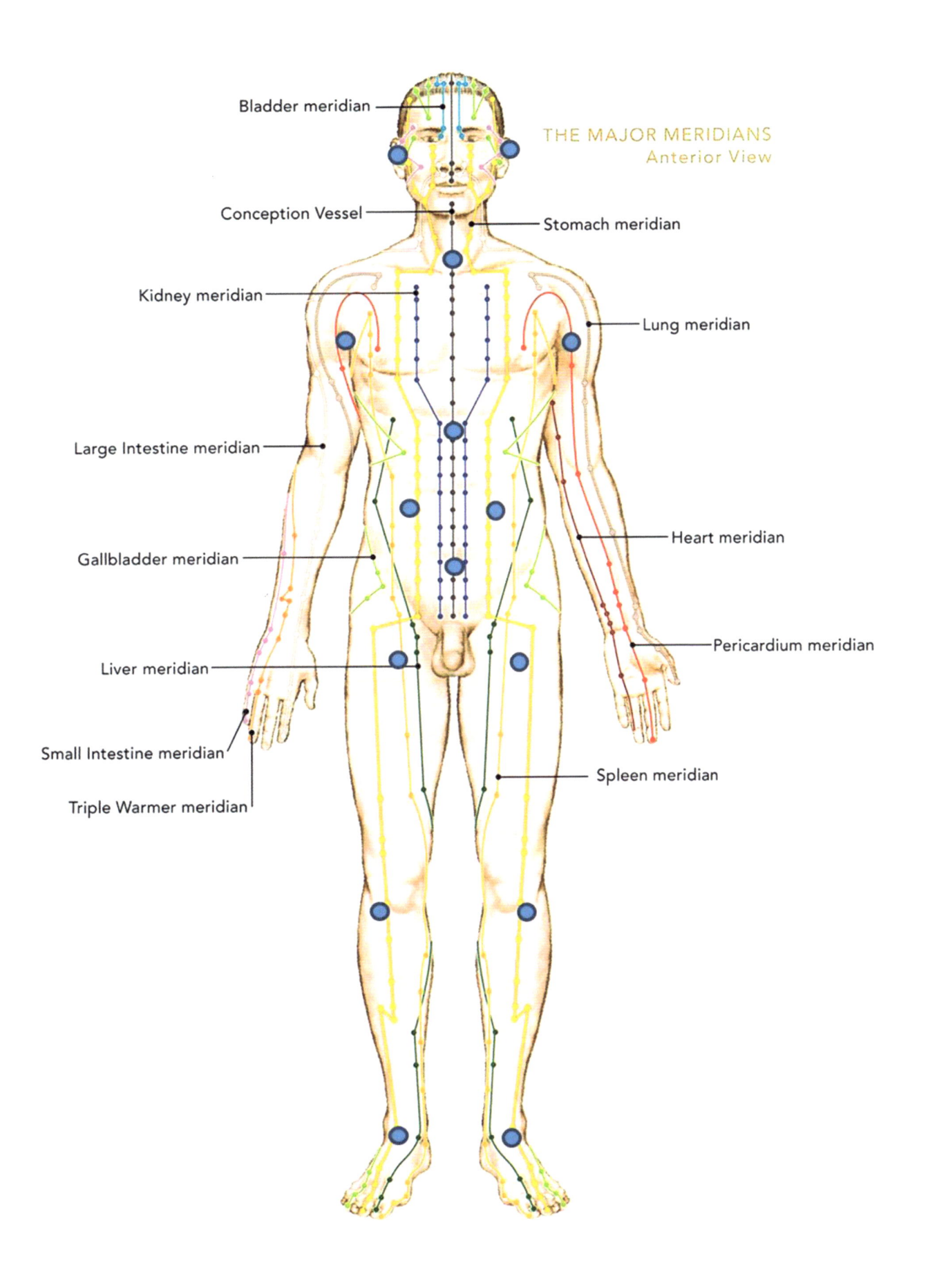

Basic Relaxation 1

Each sequence is labeled in order A, B, C, etc.
Always start with their left side

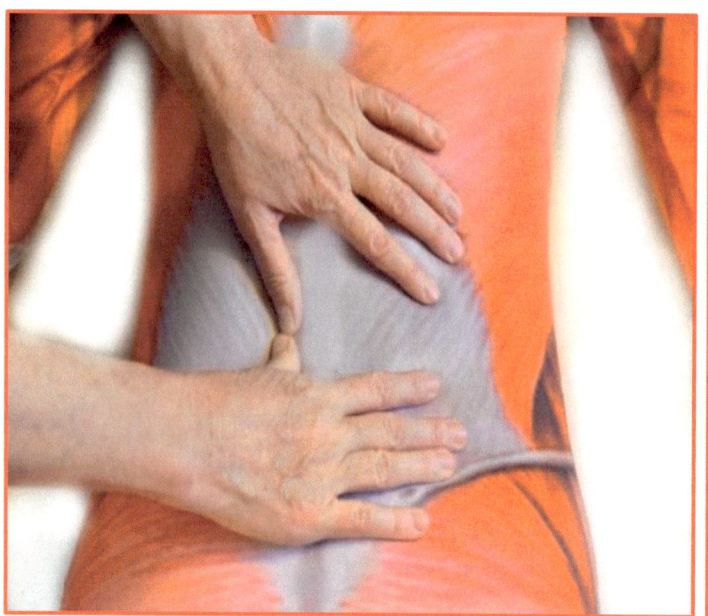

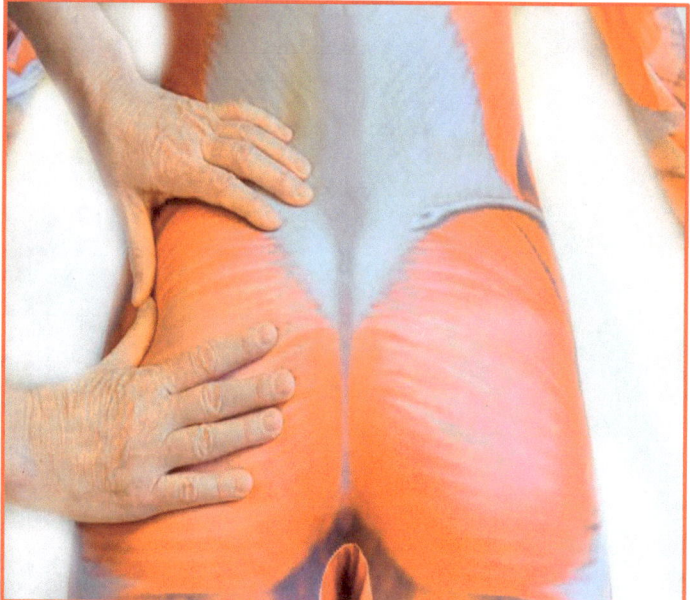

Sequence A-BRP #1

Movements 1 & 2:
Start 2 fingers above the hip line

Pull back and roll over Erector Longissimus

Movement 3:
Place fingers on top of sacrum use thumbs pull down the Gluteus Max to IT band then roll back up.

#4 Repeat on other side.

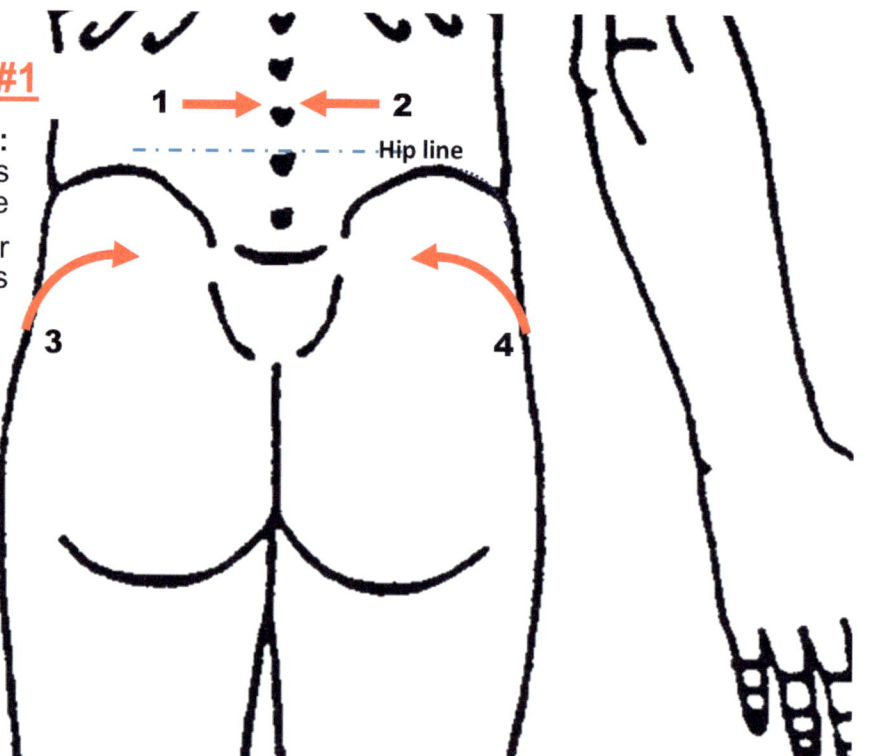

Hip line

Copyright ©2018-2022 Michelle Lally, LMBT, Ca, NCBTMB, GA, FL | Ph: 704-929-9757 | www.BowsageTherapy.com

Basic Relaxation 2

Sequence B-BRP #2

Movements 5 & 6: Reach under lateral scapula (teres attachments) and roll back up to starting point

Movements 1-4: Start 2 fingers below the Scapula line

Pull back and roll over Erector Longissimus

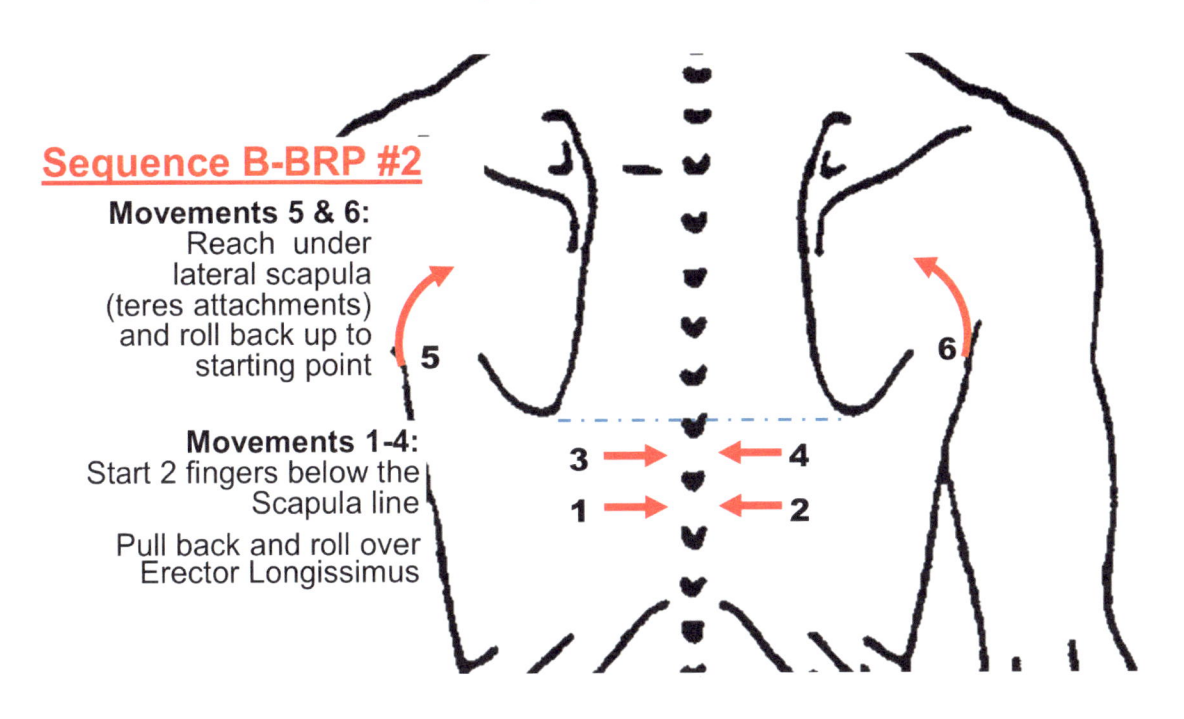

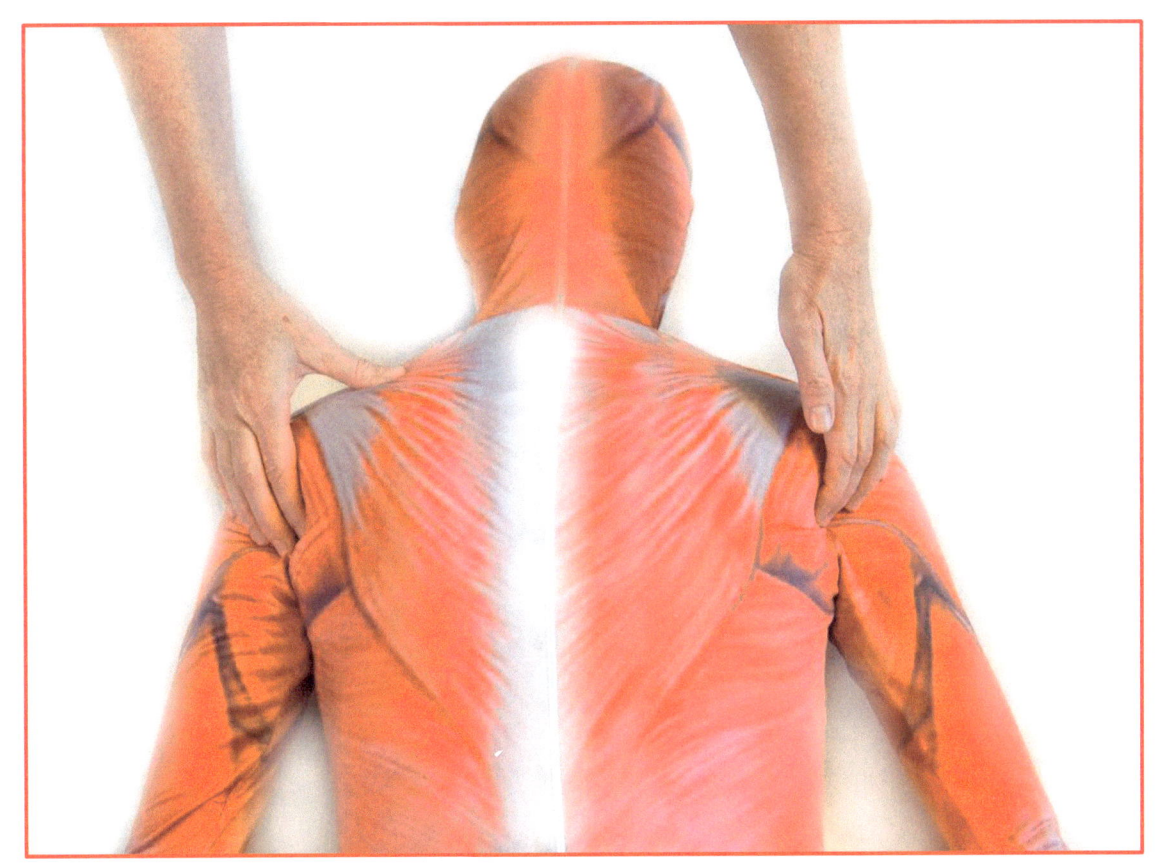

Pause and Rest

Basic Relaxation 3

Sequence A/BRP #3

Movements 1-6
1&4-Hold Tuberosity "X"

2&5 Use thubls pull down, roll up over bicep femoris

3&6 repeat-no need to hold X

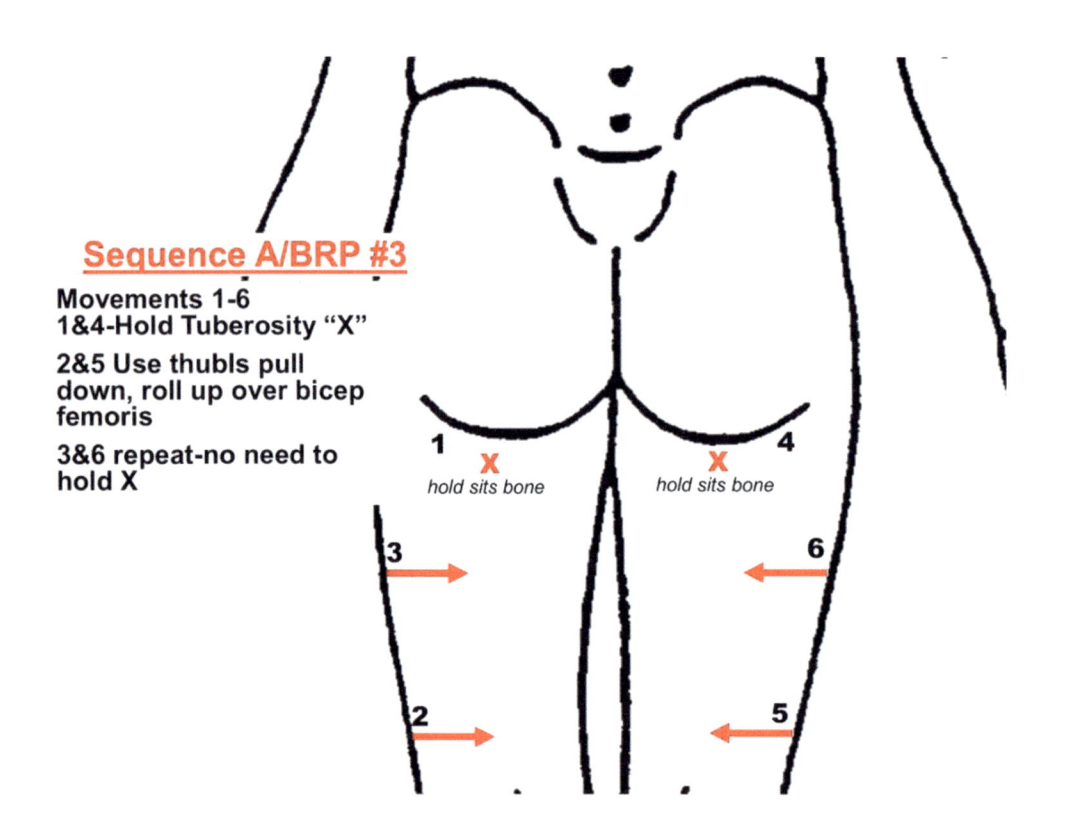

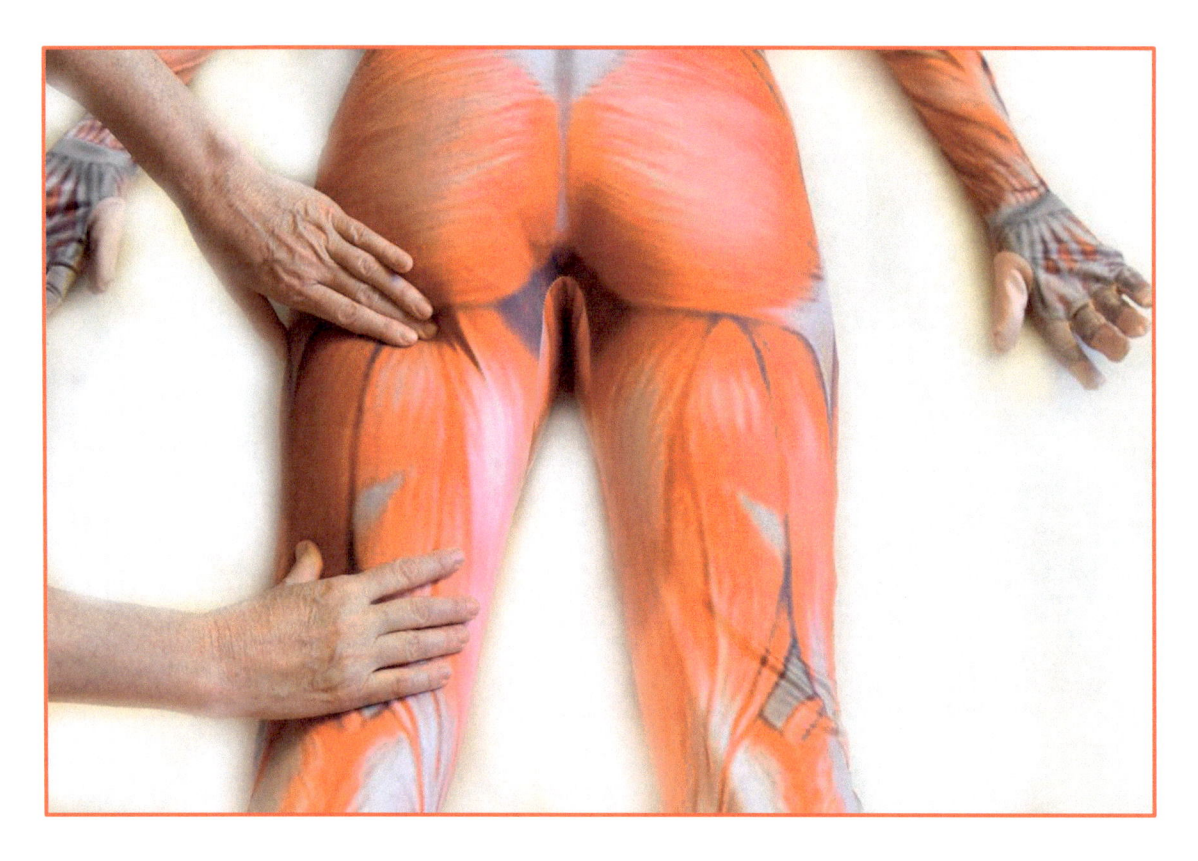

1   X hold sits bone   4   X hold sits bone

Basic Relaxation 4

Sequence B/BRP #4

**Movements 1-6:
Start at scapula line**

Pull down facia, move towards spine circle back to scapula

Pause and Rest

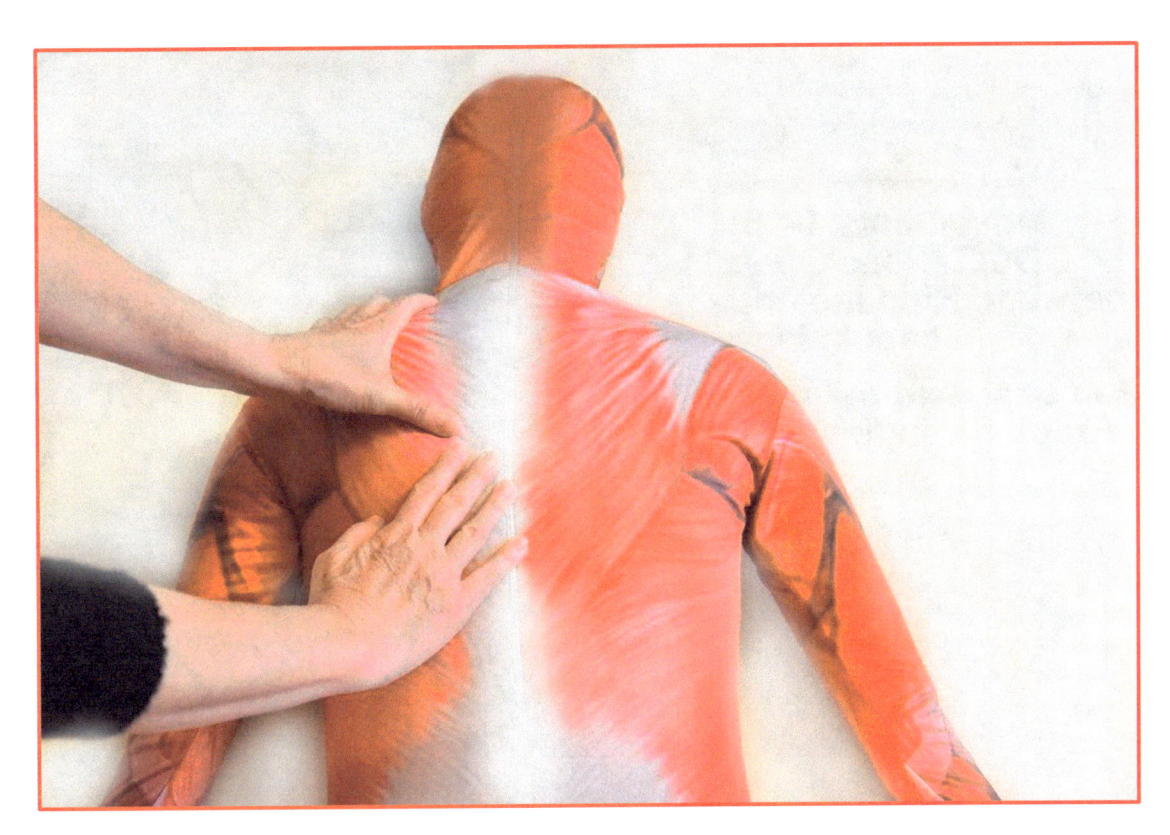

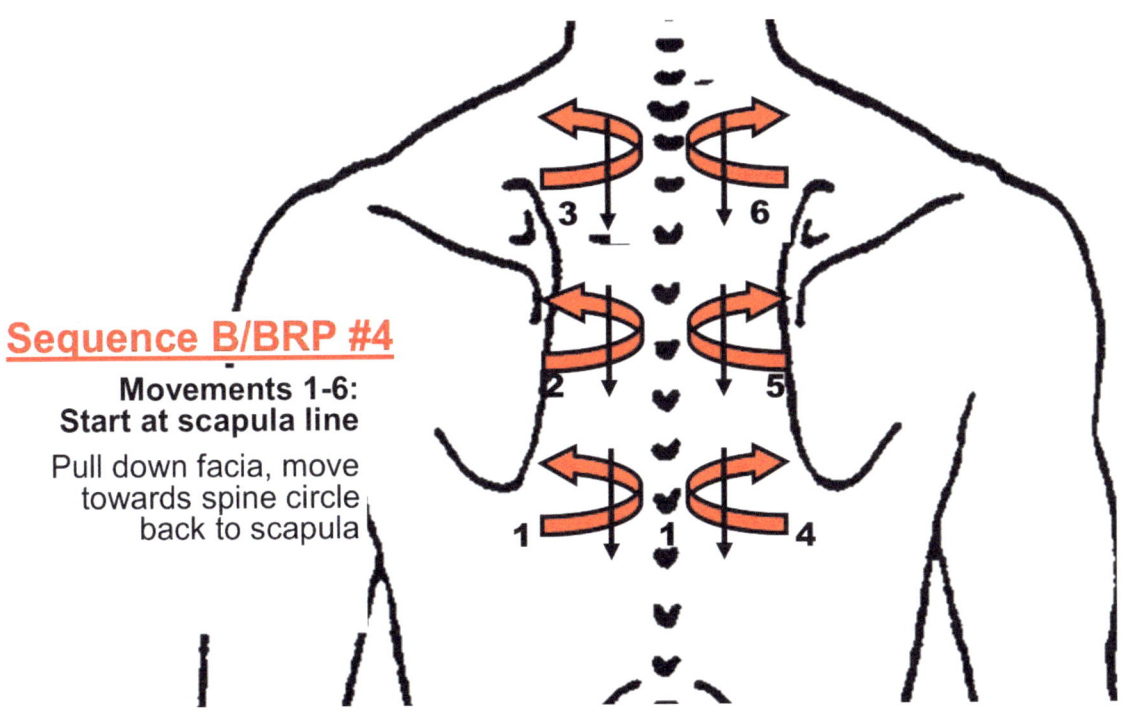

Kidney 1

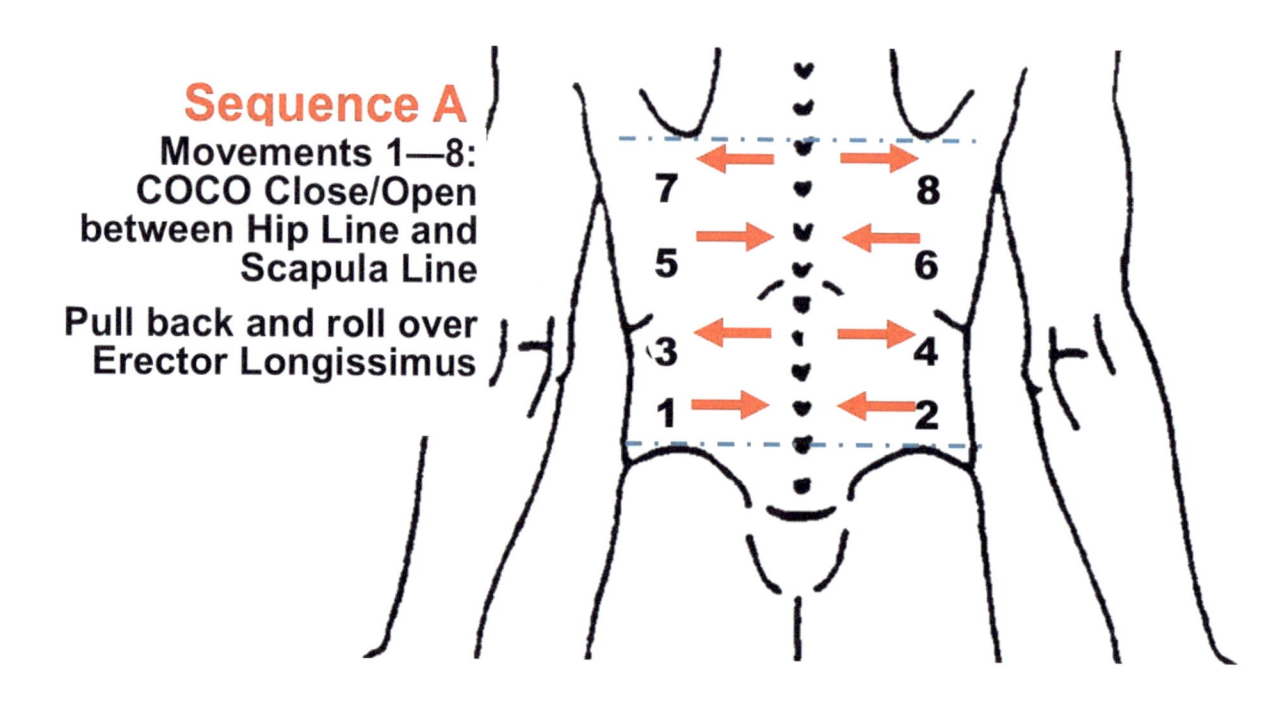

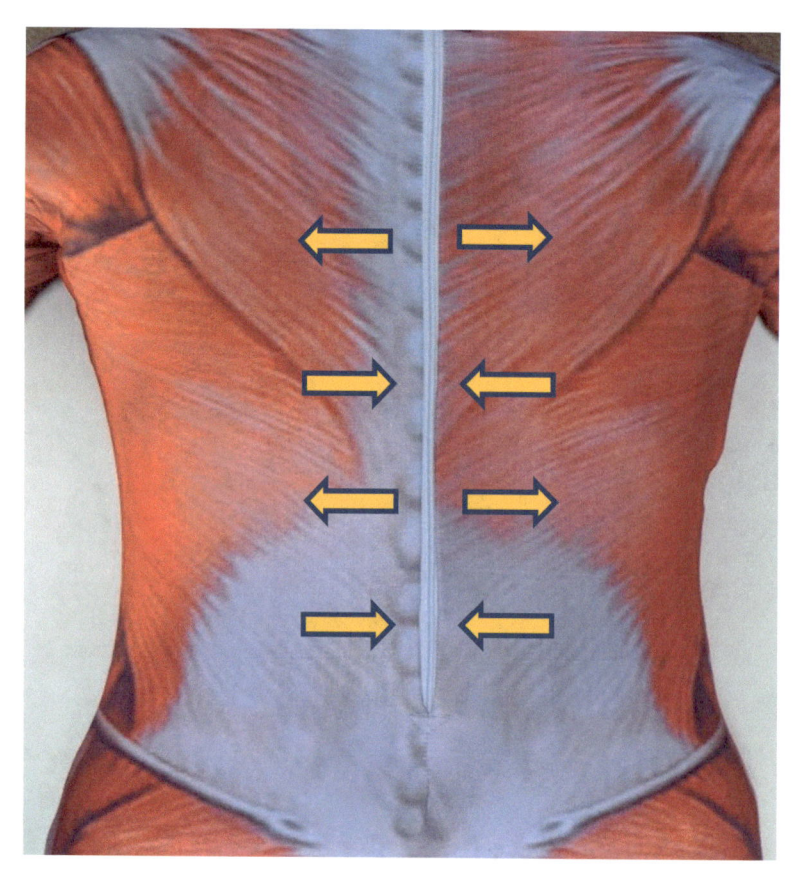

Sequence A

Movements 1—8:
COCO Close/Open between Hip Line and Scapula Line

Pull back and roll over Erector Longissimus

Hamstrings 1

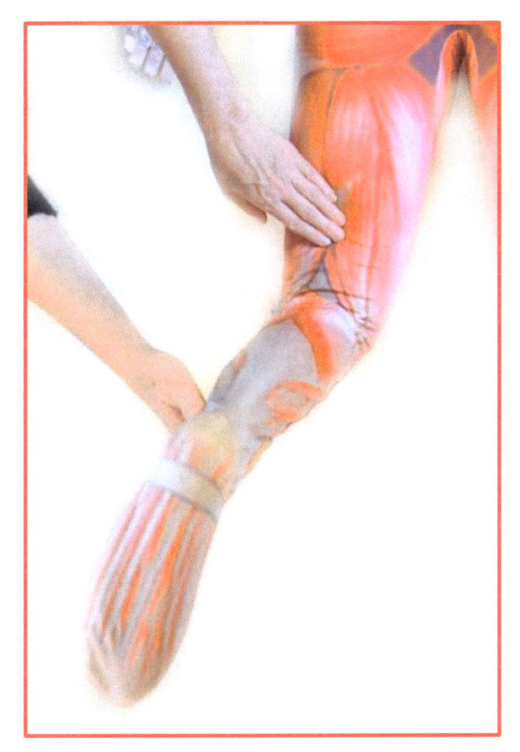

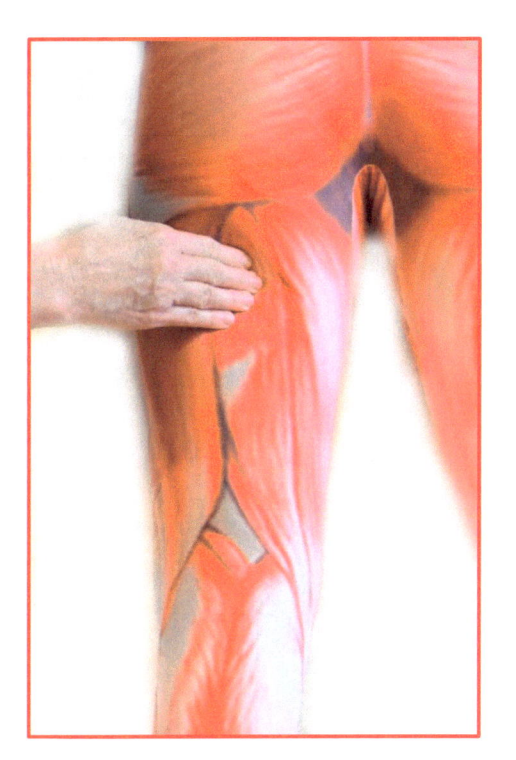

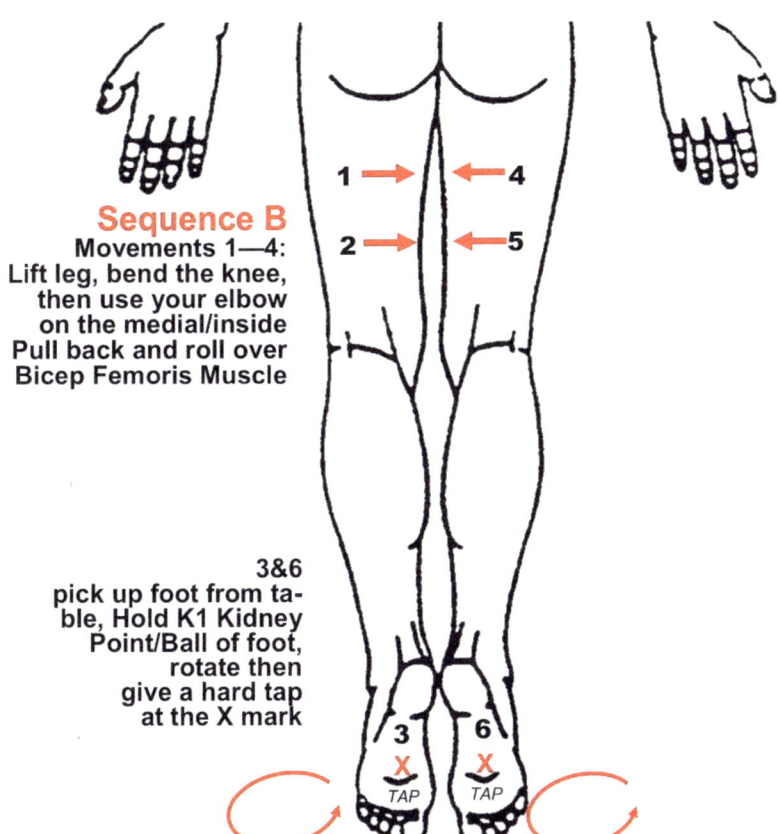

Sequence B
Movements 1—4:
Lift leg, bend the knee, then use your elbow on the medial/inside
Pull back and roll over Bicep Femoris Muscle

3 & 6
pick up foot from table, Hold K1 Kidney Point/Ball of foot, rotate then give a hard tap at the X mark

Pause & Rest

Kidney 2

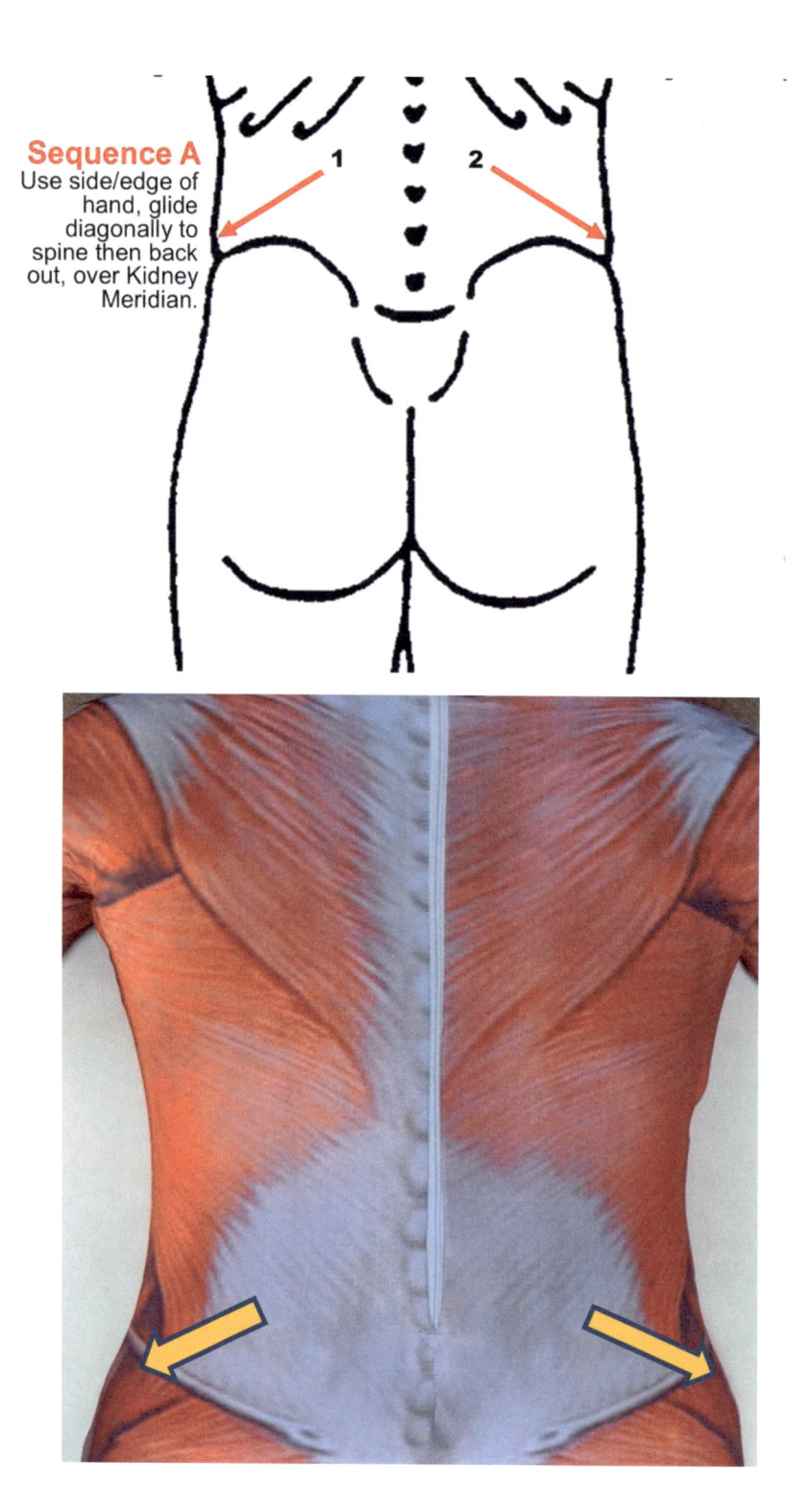

Sequence A
Use side/edge of hand, glide diagonally to spine then back out, over Kidney Meridian.

Pause and Rest

Lungs

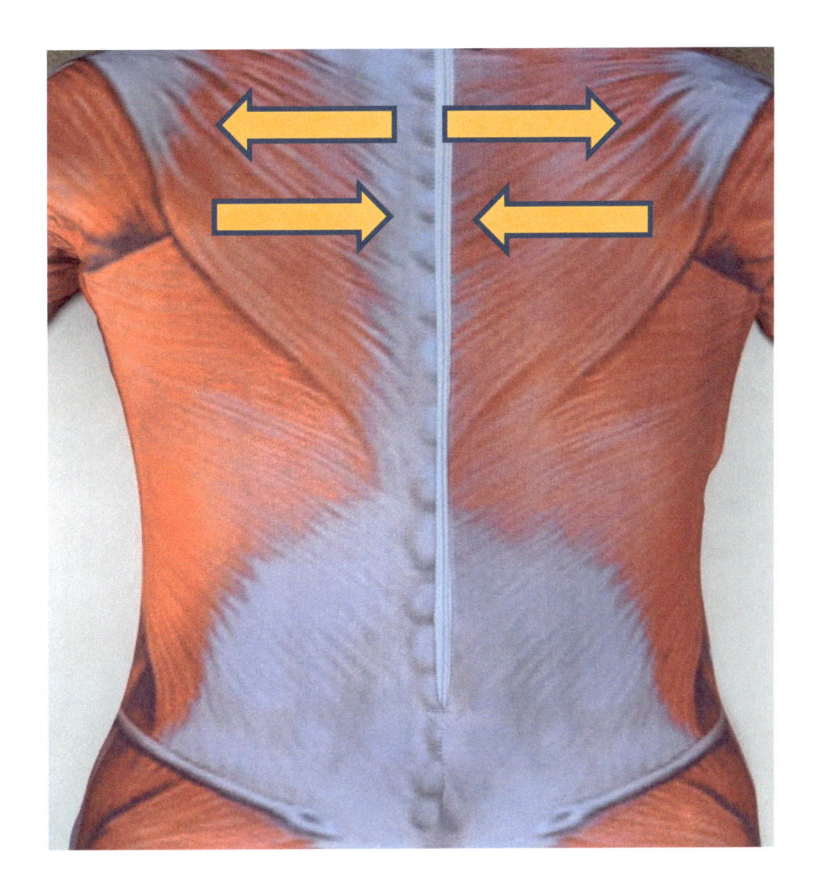

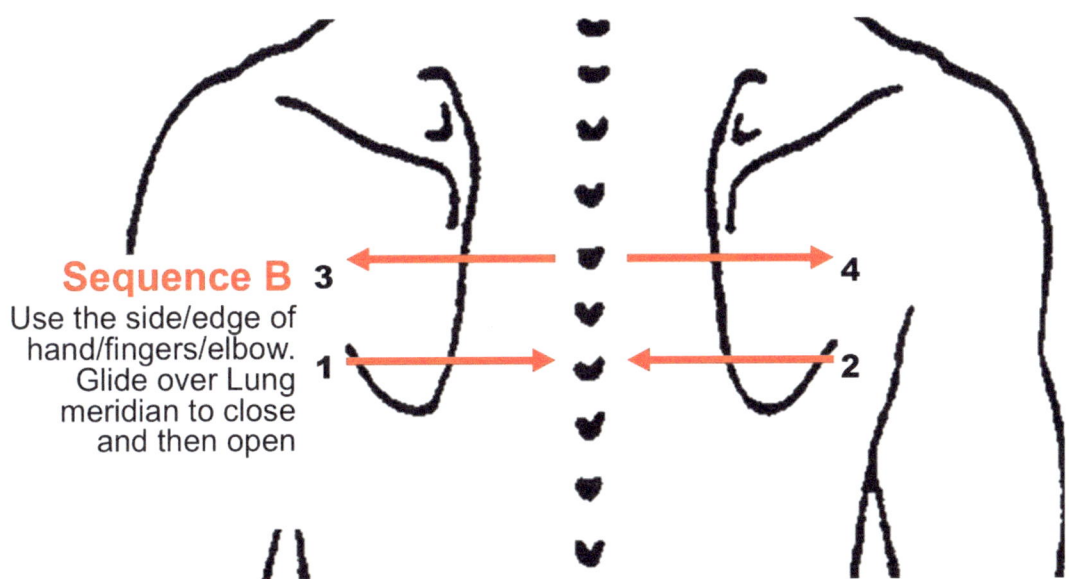

Sequence B
Use the side/edge of hand/fingers/elbow. Glide over Lung meridian to close and then open

Pause Then Turn Over

Neck 1 Sequence

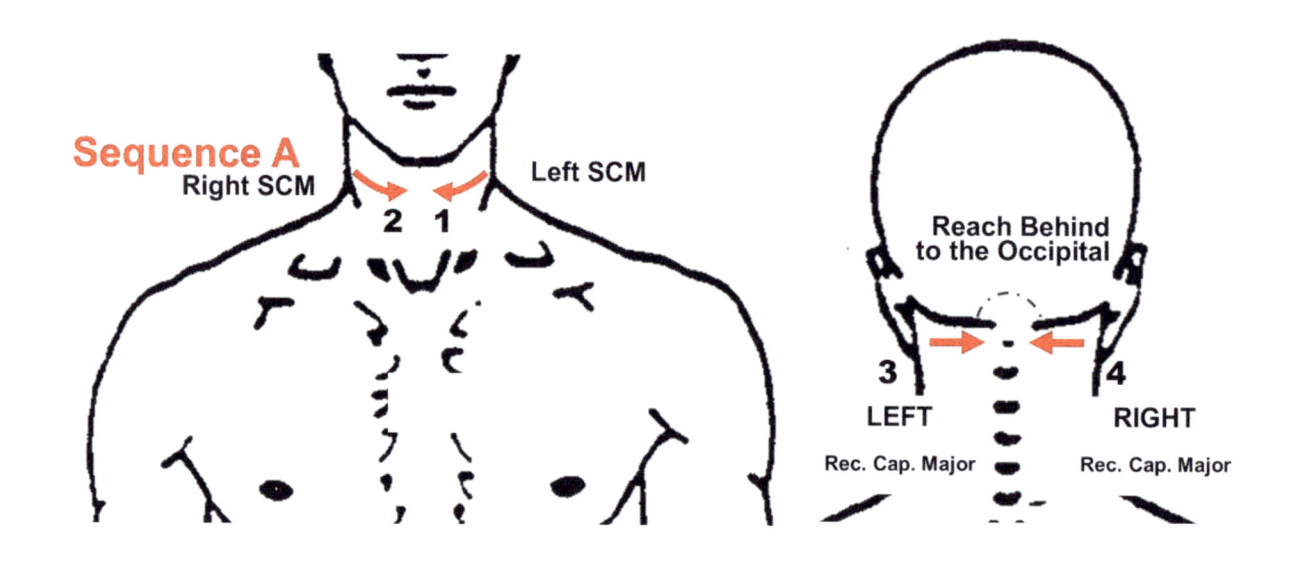

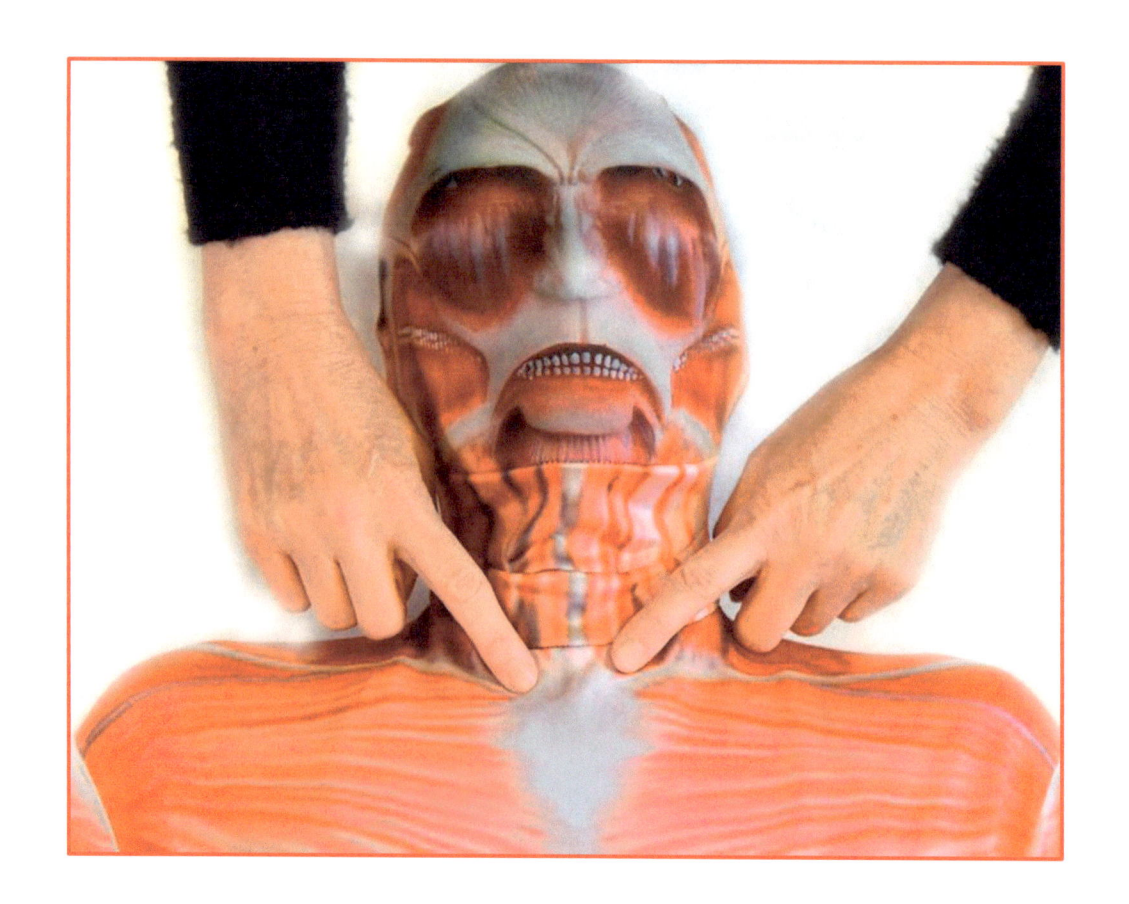

Sequence A
Right SCM — 2
Left SCM — 1

Reach Behind to the Occipital
3 LEFT — Rec. Cap. Major
4 RIGHT — Rec. Cap. Major

Copyright ©2018-2022 Michelle Lally, LMBT, Ca, NCBTMB, GA, FL | Ph: 704-929-9757 | www.BowsageTherapy.com

Diaphram

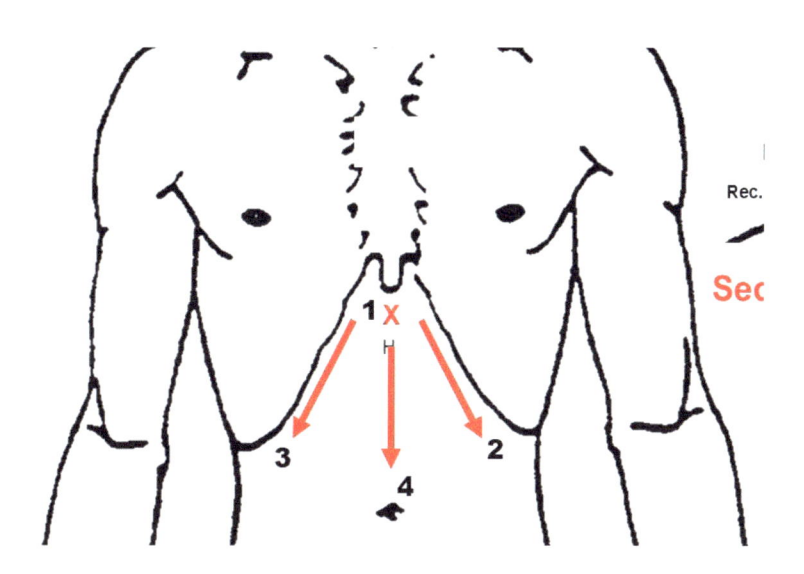

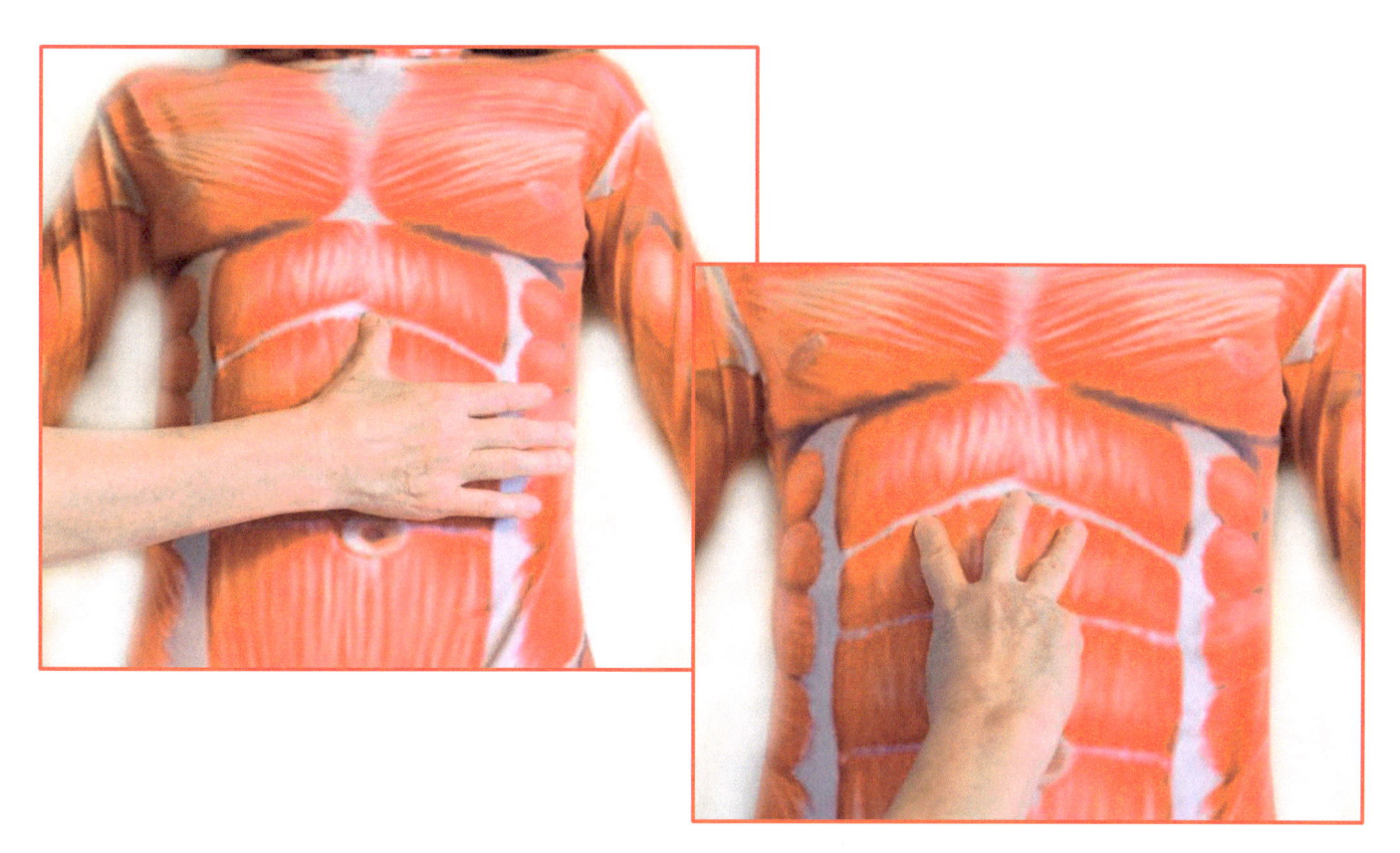

Knee 1 Sequence

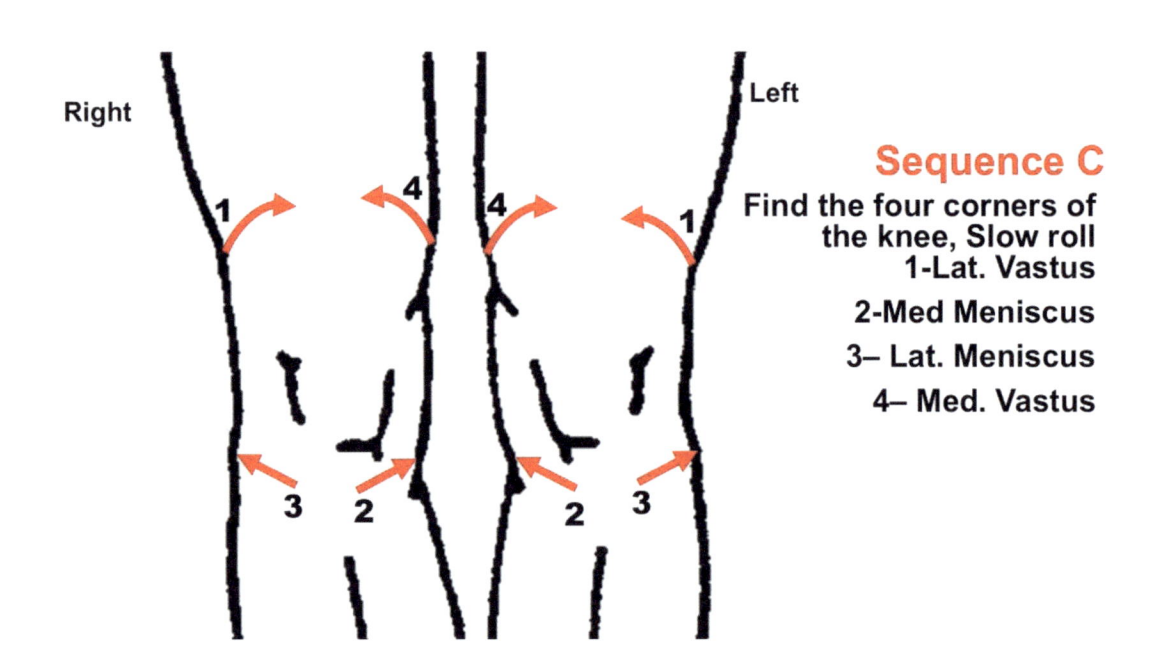

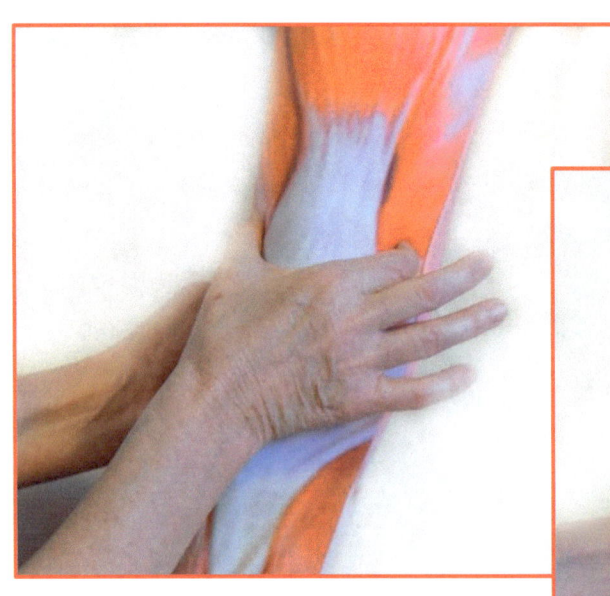

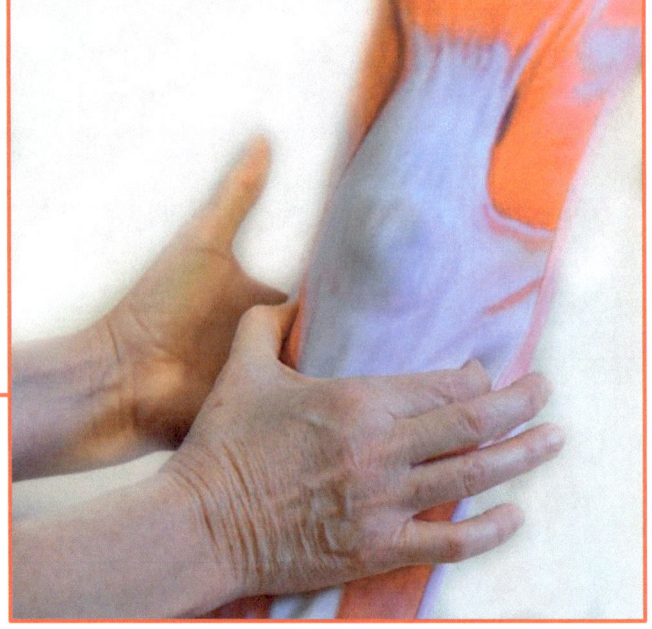

Sequence C
Find the four corners of the knee, Slow roll
1- Lat. Vastus
2- Med Meniscus
3– Lat. Meniscus
4– Med. Vastus

Pause and Rest

Neck 2 Sequence

Sequence A

Reach behind tips of fingers touching gentle pull out and roll back in over Trapezius

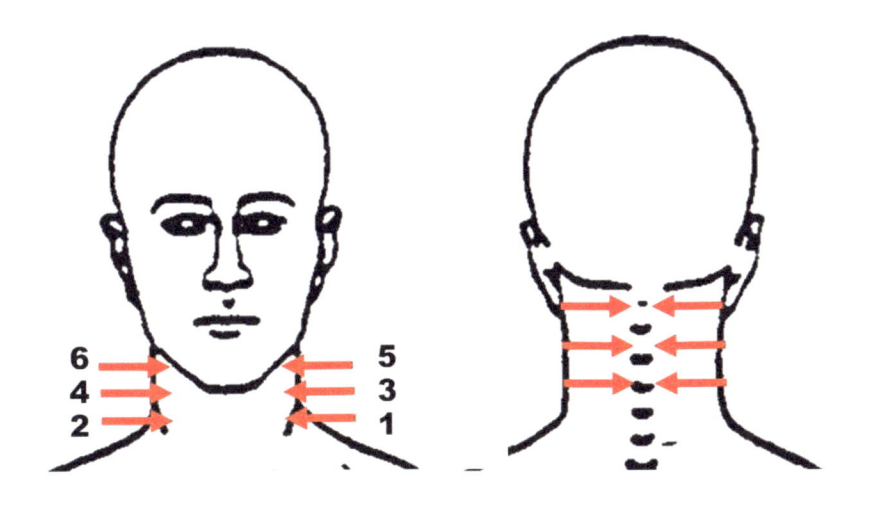

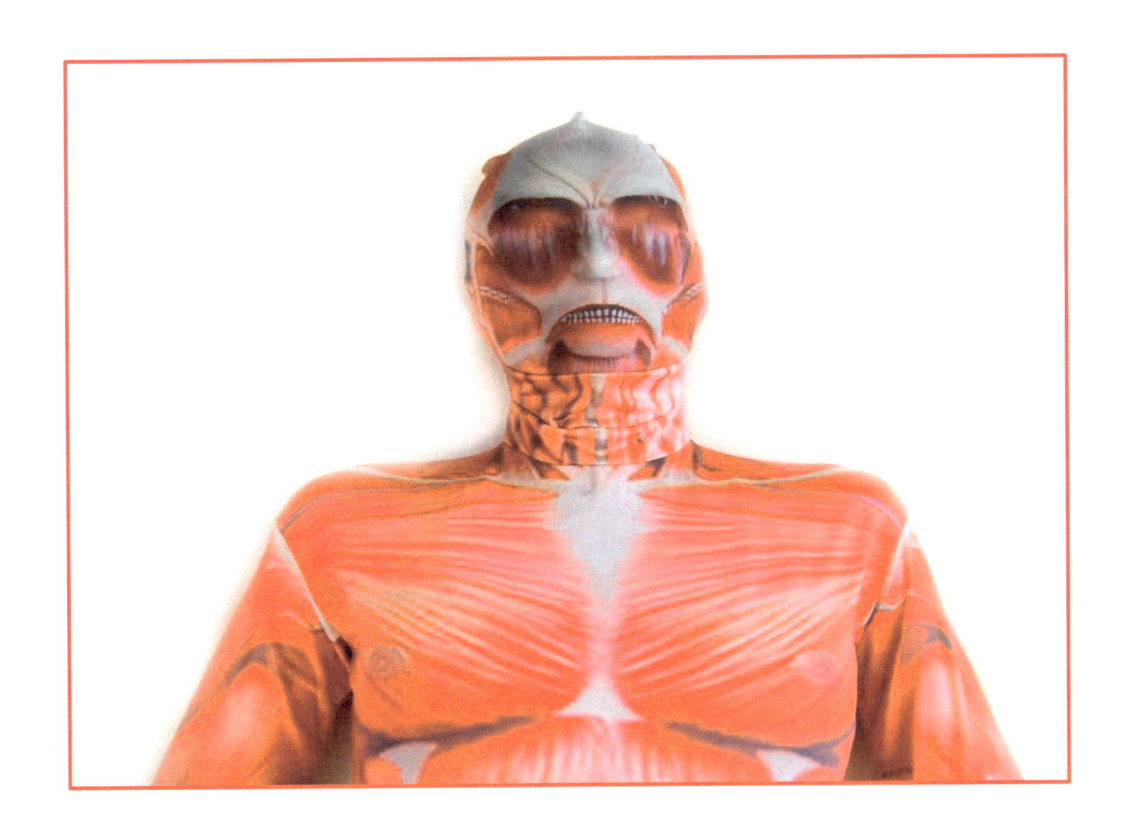

Hamstrings

Sequence B
Reach around/under outer thigh push into the middle, lift up, pull to open, bend knee, support foot, continue to open the calf.

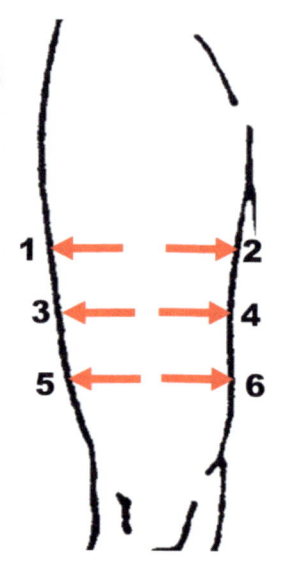

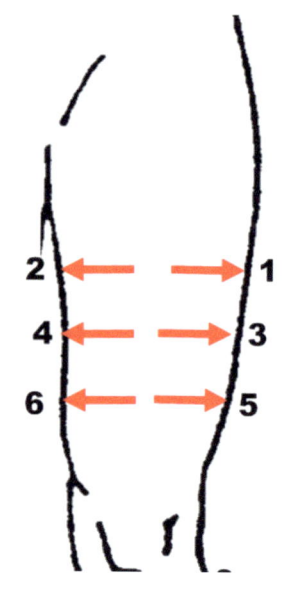

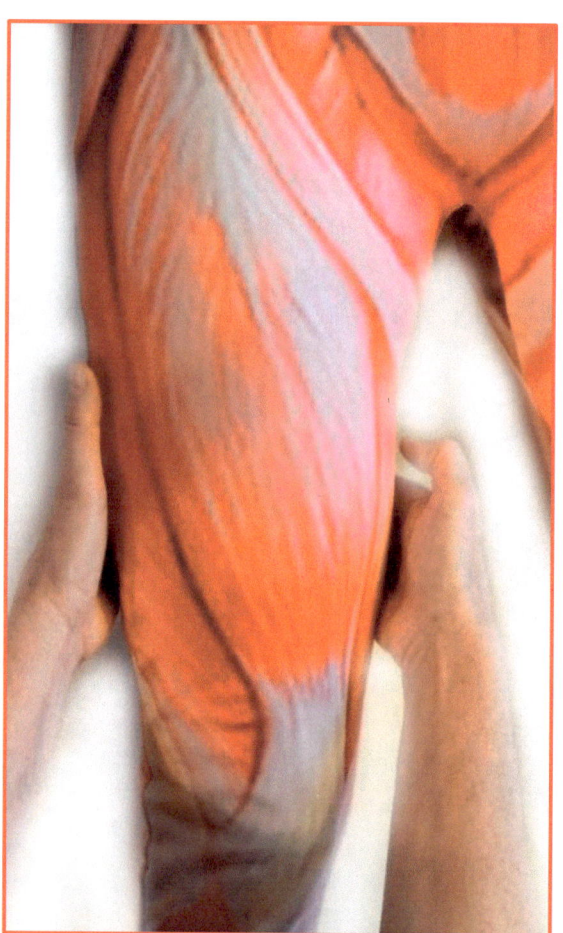

Caf and Achilles

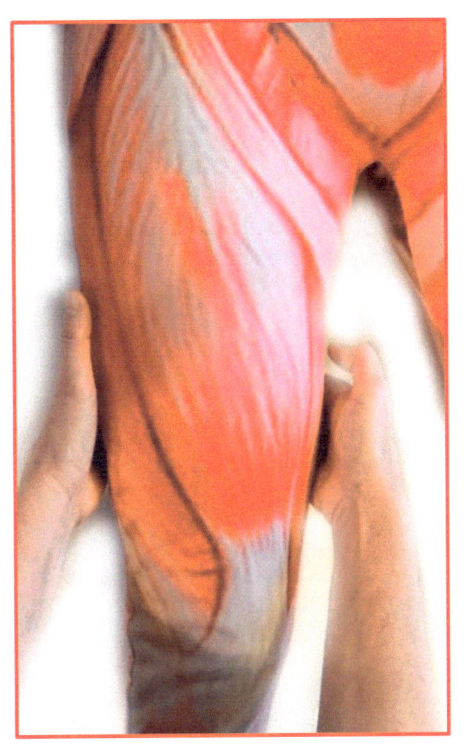

Sequence C

1-5 Reach around to back of calf, gently push in both hands together, pull to open, at same time 5 times.

6-8 medial to lateral over Achilles.

9 reach behind and gently pull forward over the soleus

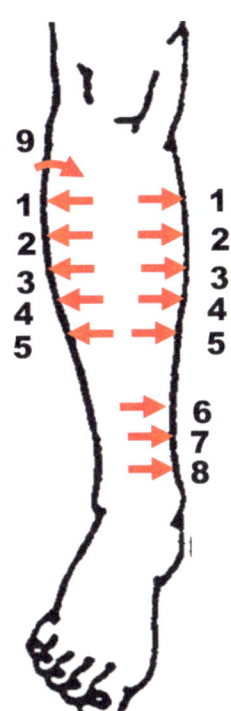

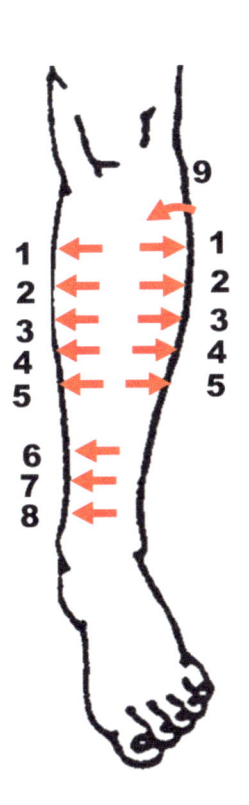

Pause and Rest

Knee 3 & Pelvis

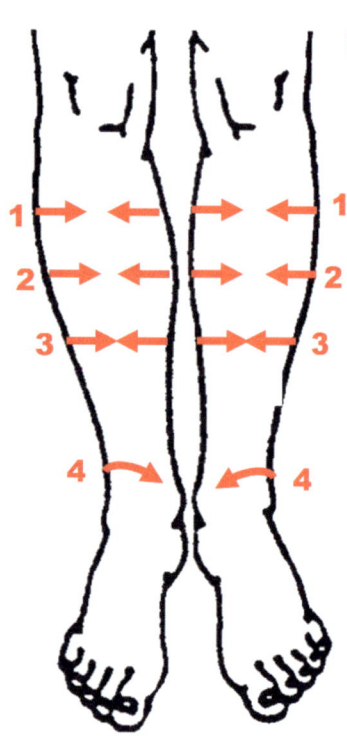

Sequence A
Calf/Achilles

1-3 Close calf start in the middle of calf, pull out then close back to center.
4-Start at medial posterior ankle, pull lateral and back to medial

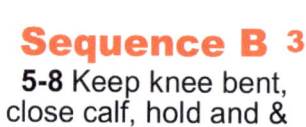

Sequence B
5-8 Keep knee bent, close calf, hold and & support **Itsy Bitsy Spider**, raise leg to engage inguinal ligament straighten leg and engage hamstring to reset hips and hamstring

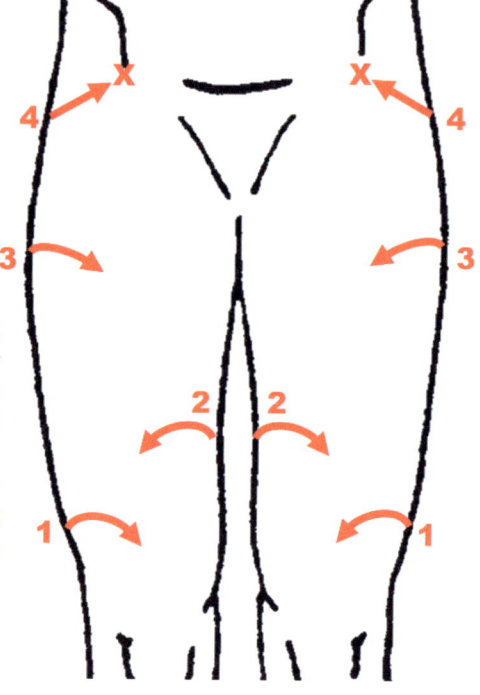

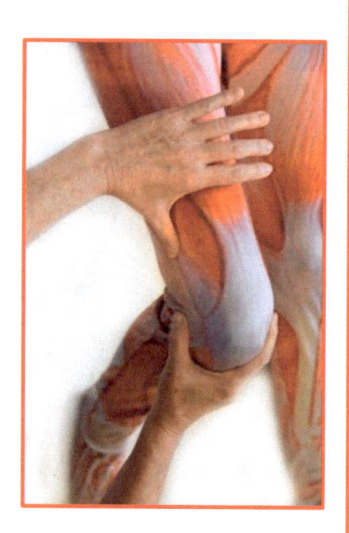

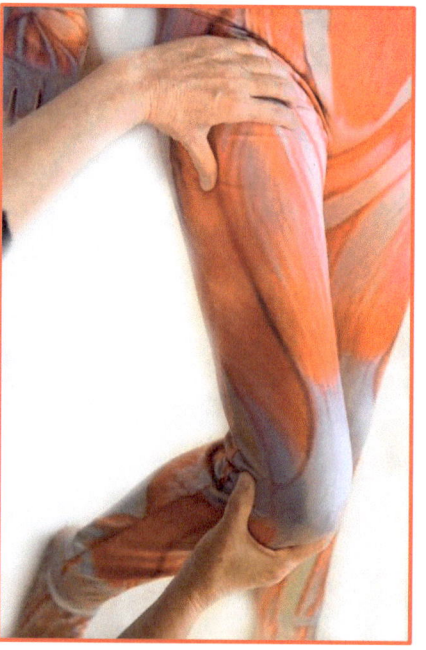

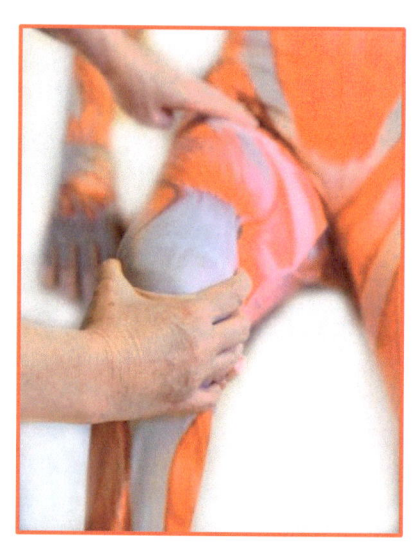

Respiratory | Allergy

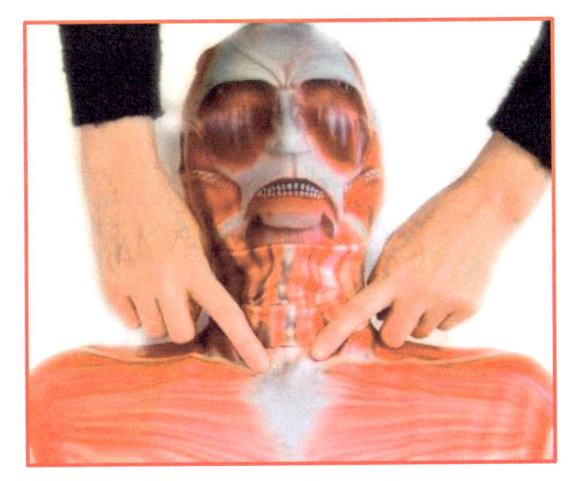

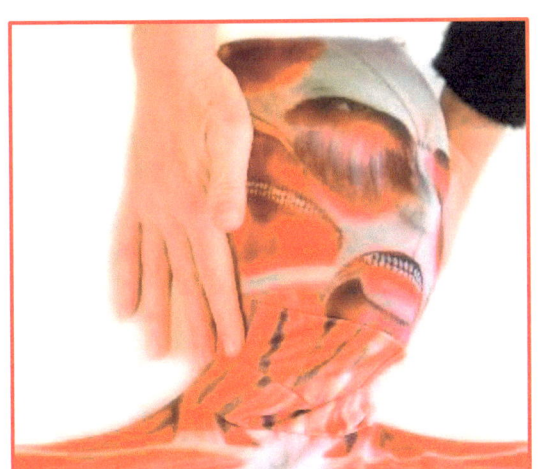

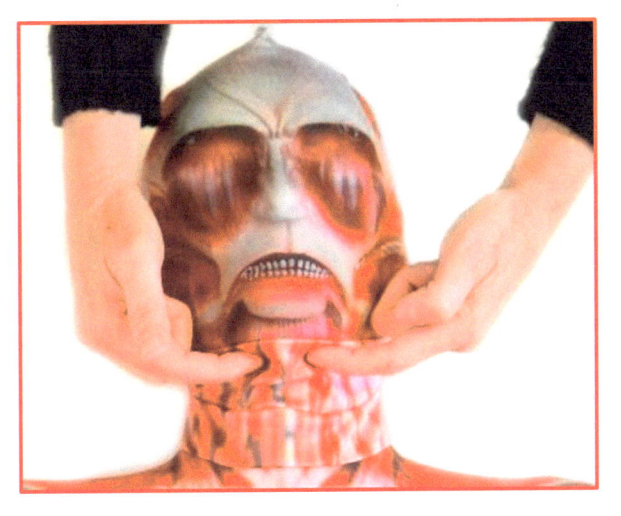

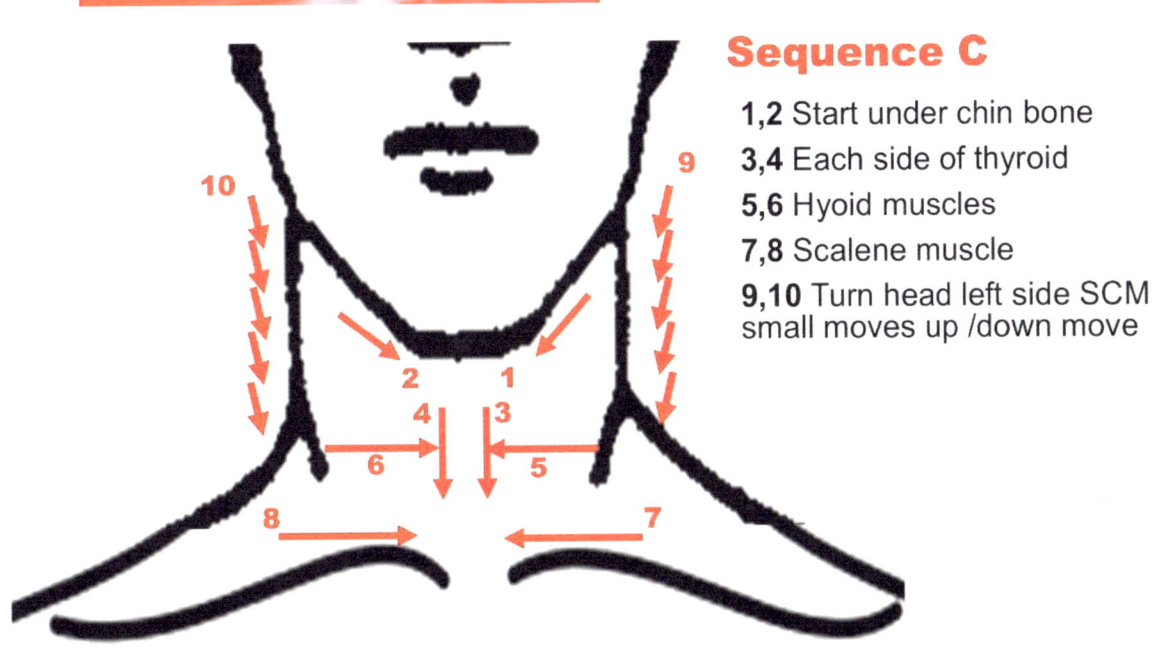

Sequence C

1,2 Start under chin bone
3,4 Each side of thyroid
5,6 Hyoid muscles
7,8 Scalene muscle
9,10 Turn head left side SCM small moves up /down move

Pause and Rest

TMJ Sequence

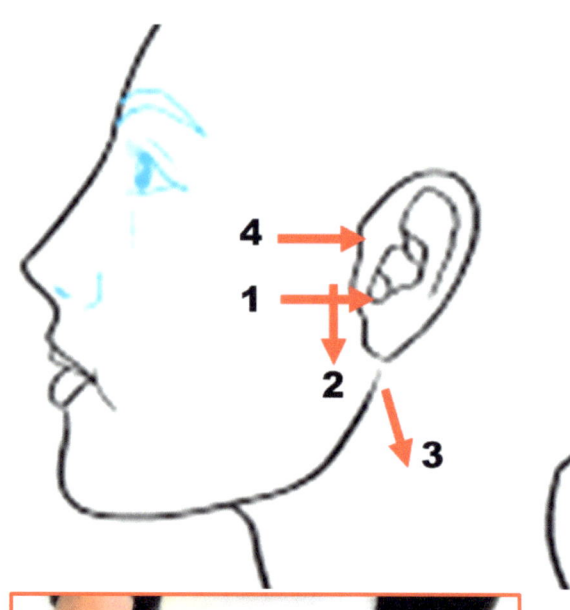

Sequence A

TMJ left then right

1-1 pterygoid away from ear then back

2-2 pterygoid up then down

3-3 Digastric up then down

4-4 temporal away from ear hen back

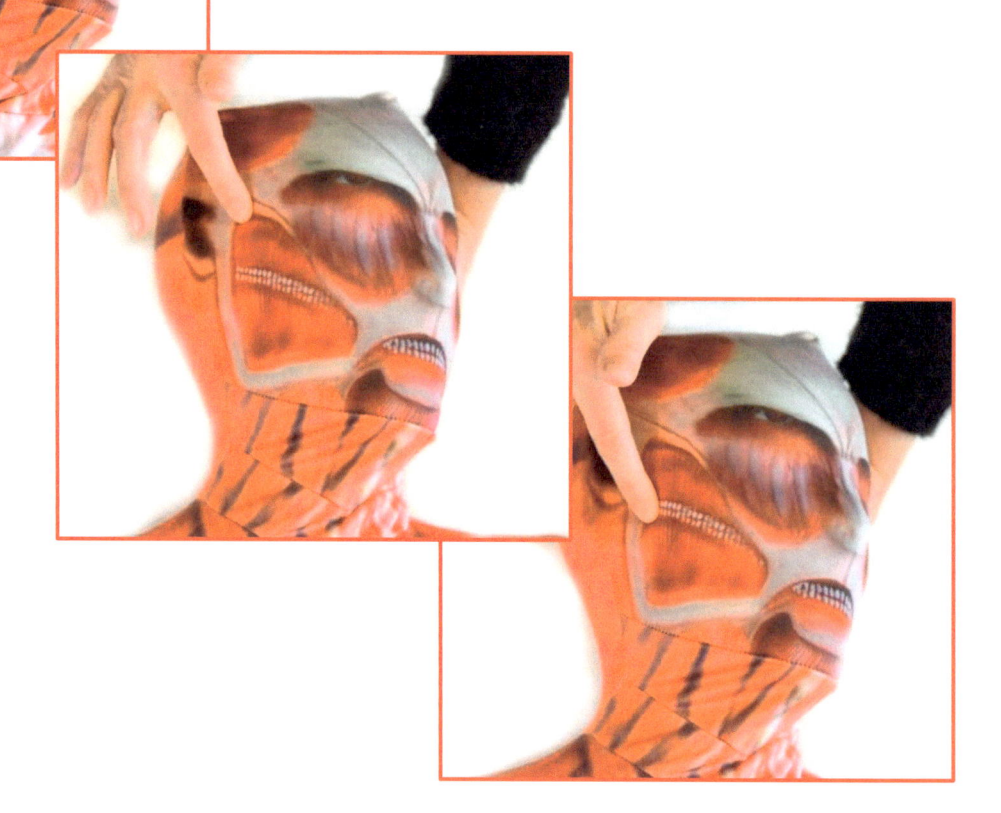

Pectoral
Sequence B

Pectoralis Major:

1-2 Upper Pec– Left hand face away from breast.

3-4 Lower Pec– Right hand face away from breast

5-6 stand at head start at top of shoulder move down under pec then roll back up

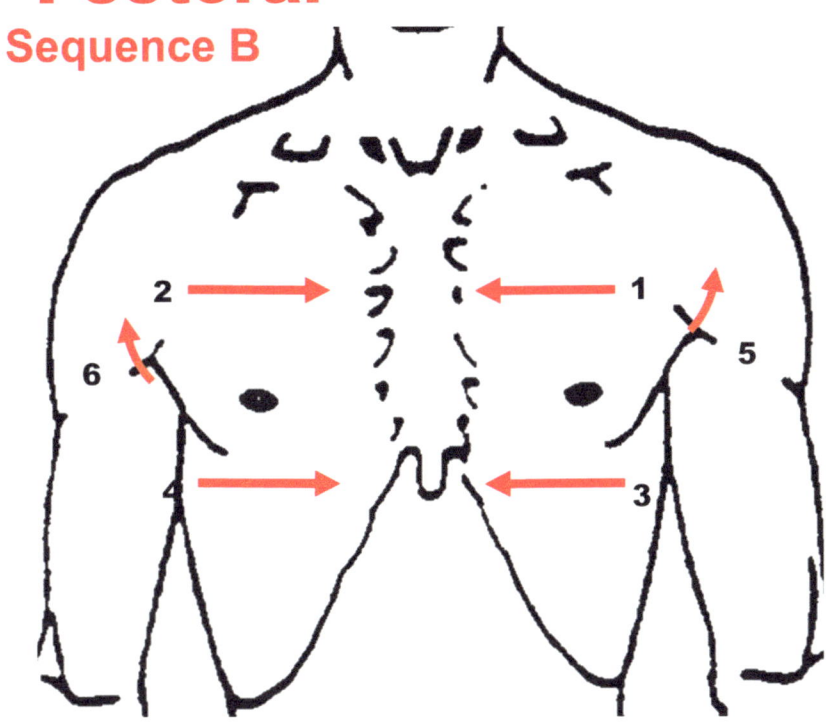

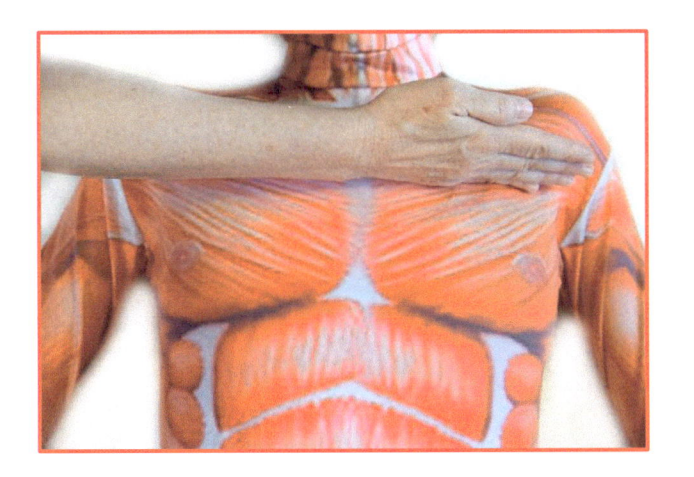

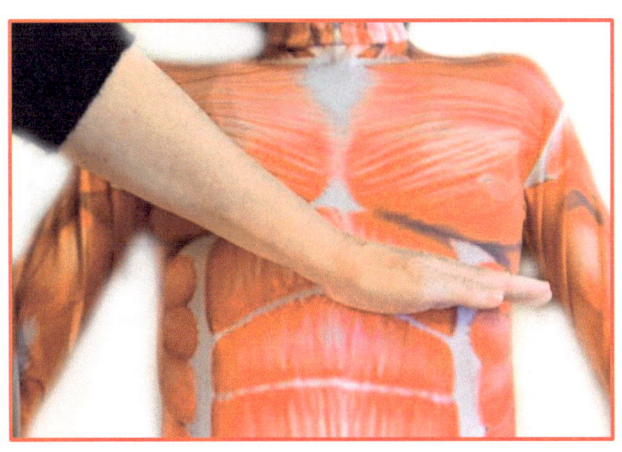

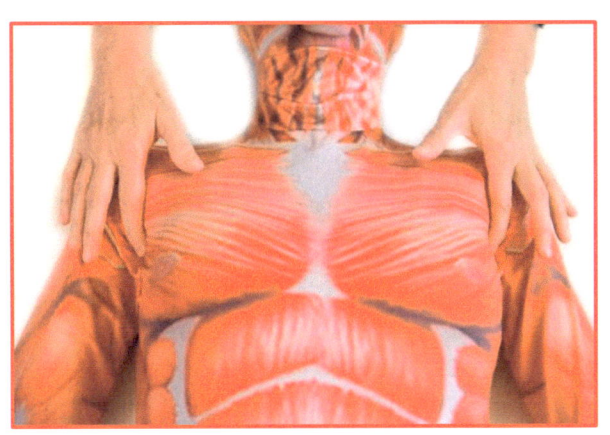

Ankle & Foot Sequence

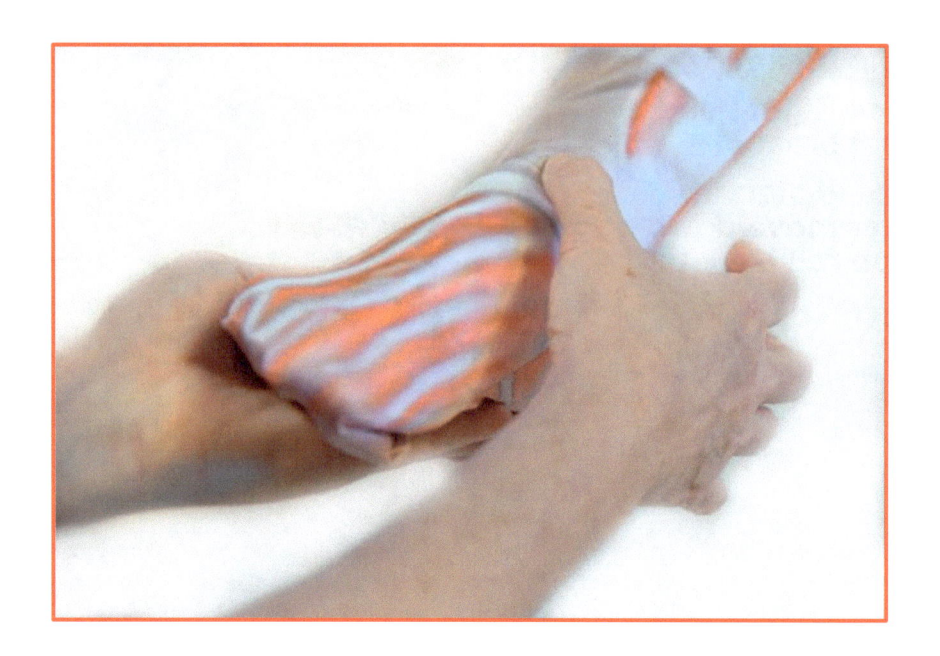

Sequence C

1 superior extensor- start medial across top then back

2 superior peroneal– start below move up then back down

3 Tibullus tendon– start below move up then back down

4 raise leg holding calf, Hold pressure on X- K1 point- rotate and tap –REPEAT ON RIGHT SIDE

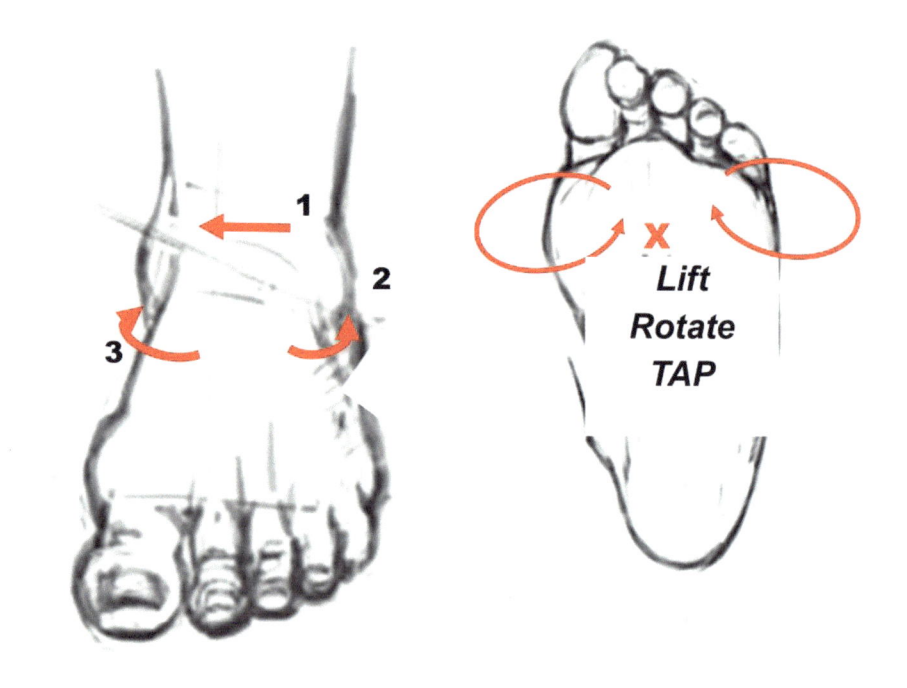

Rest and Assist

95% of the
Bowen Moves are done over the Meridian System

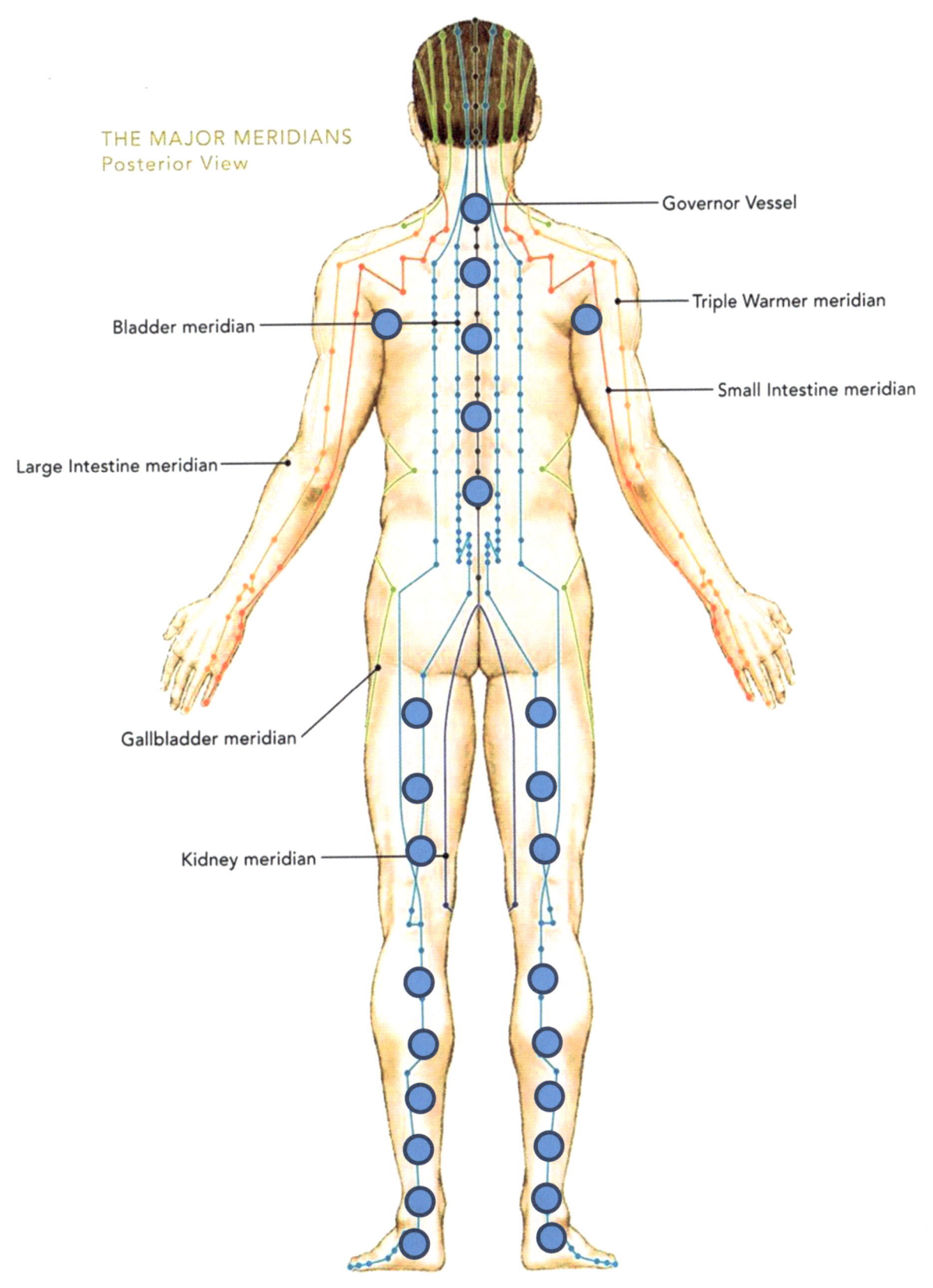

THE MAJOR MERIDIANS
Posterior View

- Governor Vessel
- Triple Warmer meridian
- Bladder meridian
- Small Intestine meridian
- Large Intestine meridian
- Gallbladder meridian
- Kidney meridian

Copyright ©2018-2022 Michelle Lally, LMBT, Ca, NCBTMB, GA, FL | Ph: 704-929-9757 | www.BowsageTherapy.com

THE MAJOR MERIDIANS
Anterior View

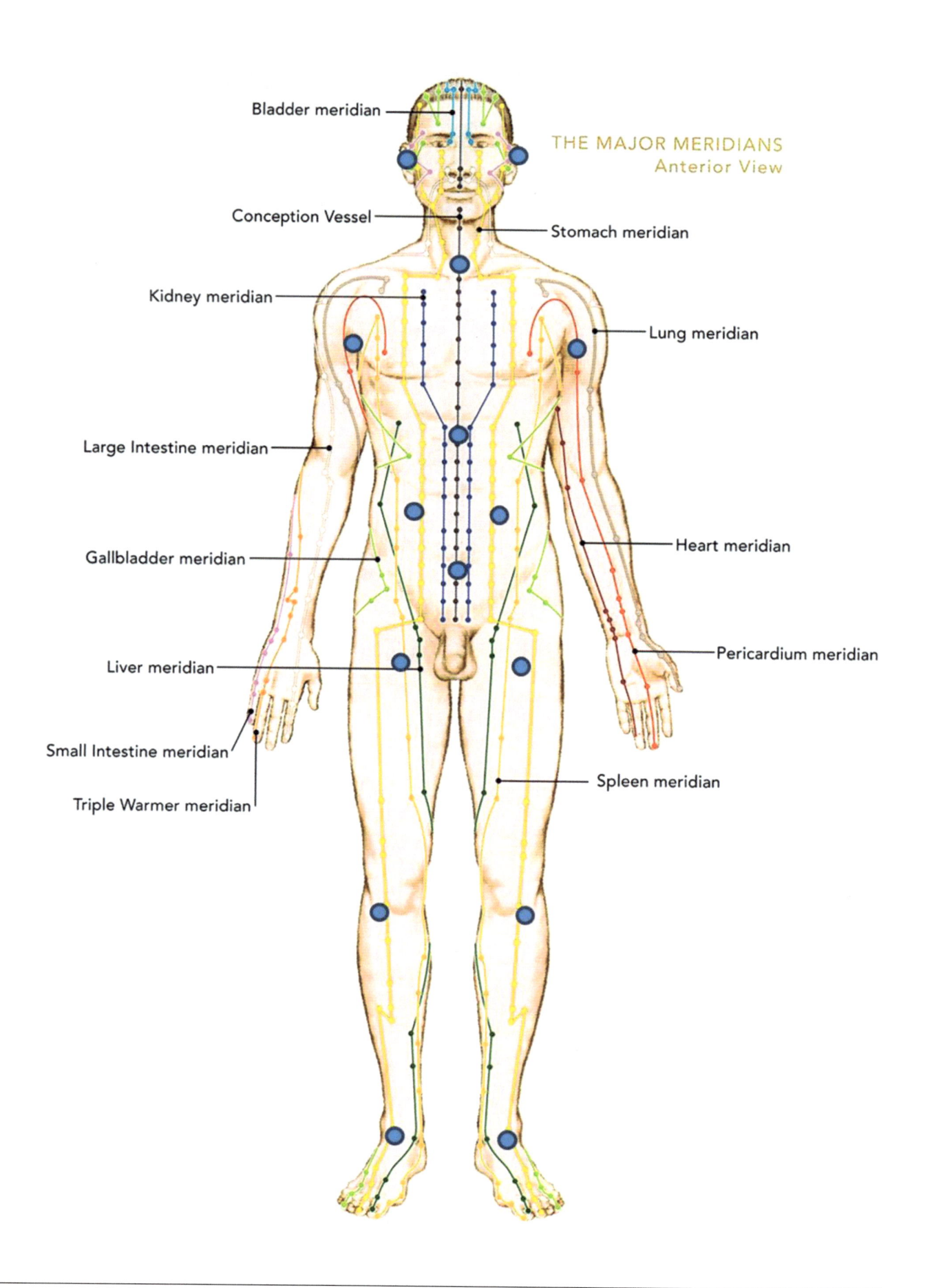

- Bladder meridian
- Conception Vessel
- Stomach meridian
- Kidney meridian
- Lung meridian
- Large Intestine meridian
- Heart meridian
- Gallbladder meridian
- Pericardium meridian
- Liver meridian
- Small Intestine meridian
- Spleen meridian
- Triple Warmer meridian

Copyright ©2018-2022 Michelle Lally, LMBT, Ca, NCBTMB, GA, FL | Ph: 704-929-9757 | www.BowsageTherapy.com

Basic Relaxation 1 and 2

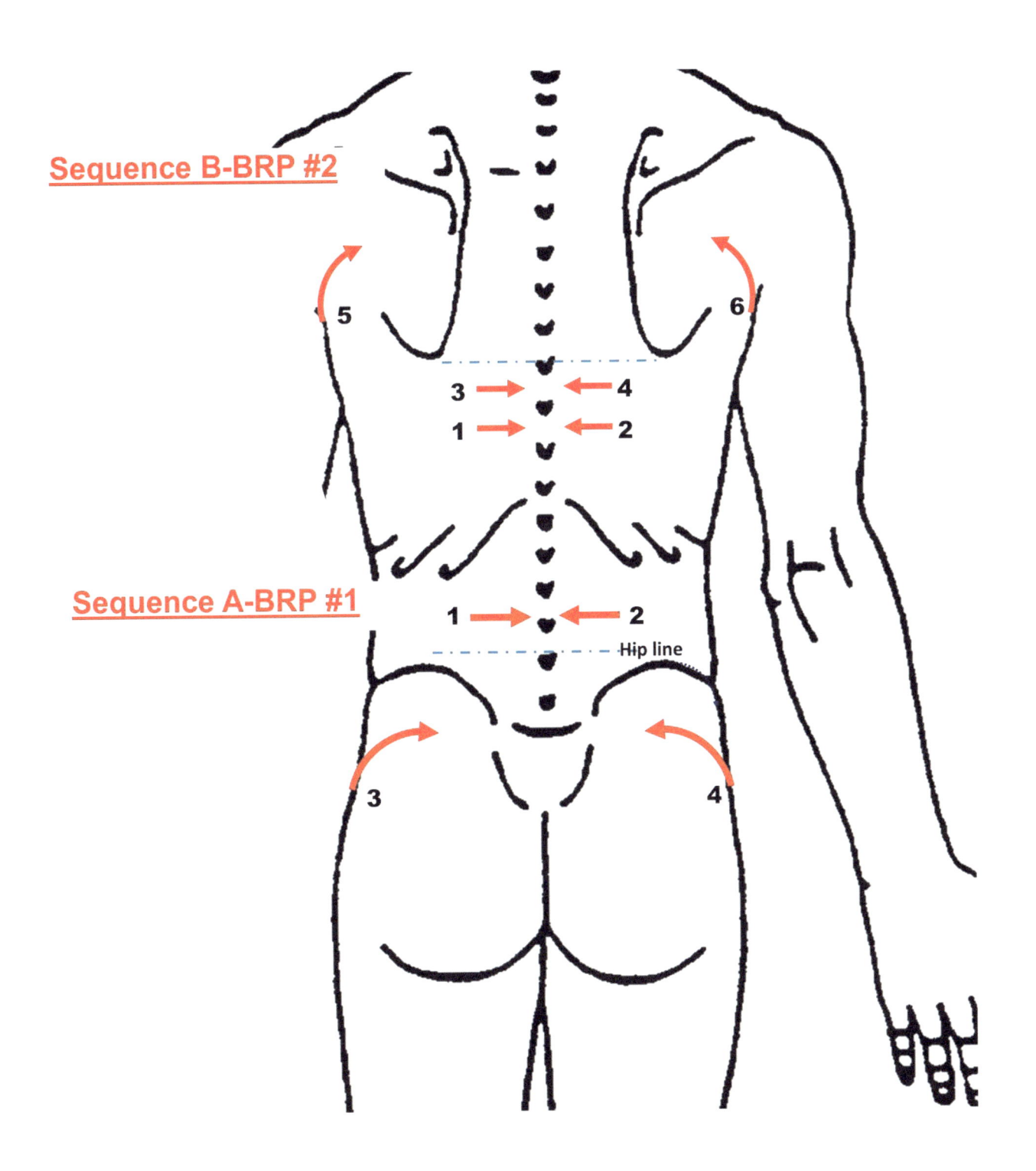

Sequence B-BRP #2

Sequence A-BRP #1

Hip line

Pause and Rest

Basic Relaxation 3 and 4

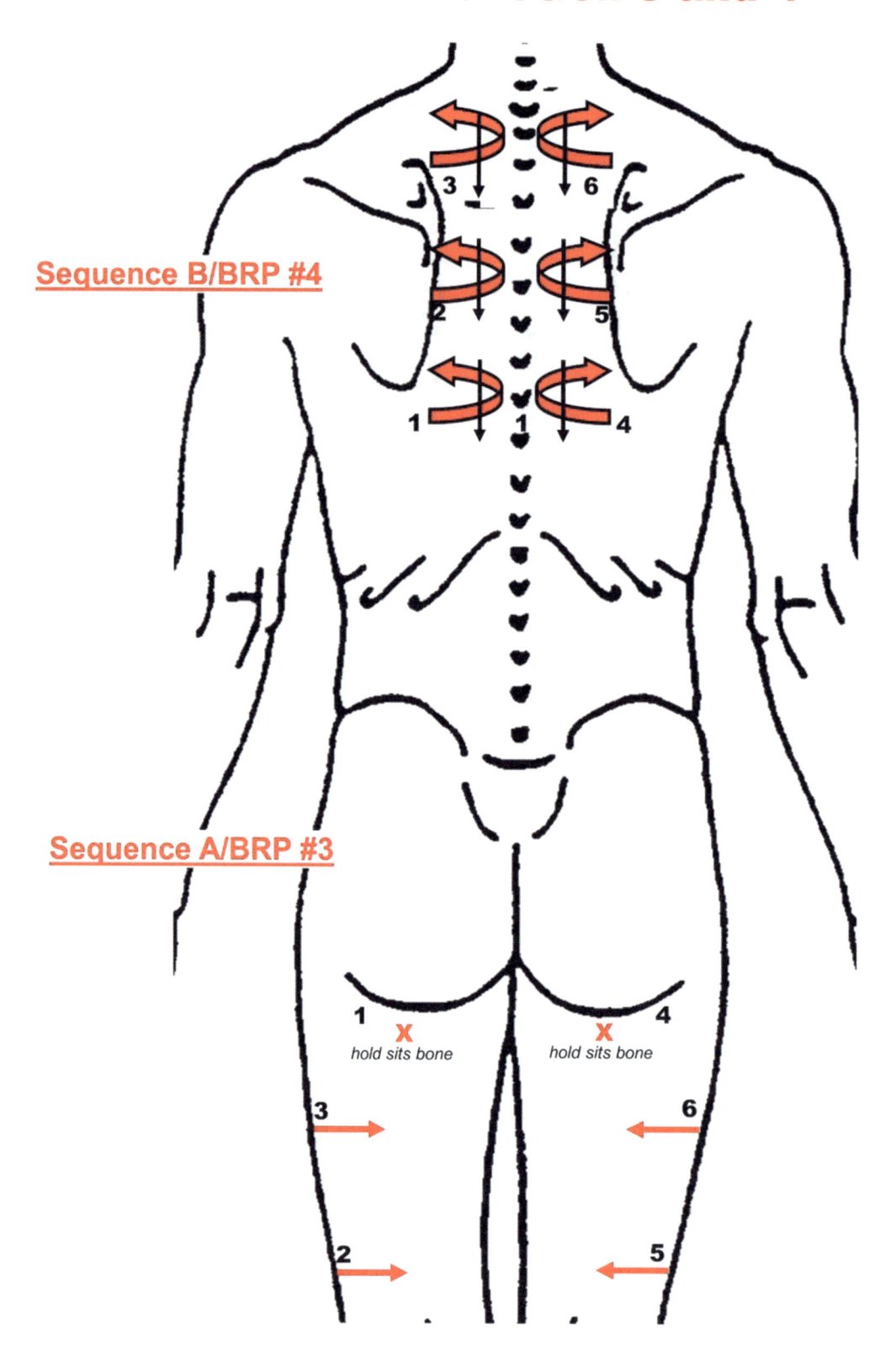

Sequence B/BRP #4

Sequence A/BRP #3

hold sits bone

hold sits bone

Pause and Rest

Kidney and Hamstring Sequences

Sequence A

C-O-C-O
Close-Open-Close-Open

7 ← → 8
5 → ← 6
3 ← → 4
1 → ← 2

Sequence B

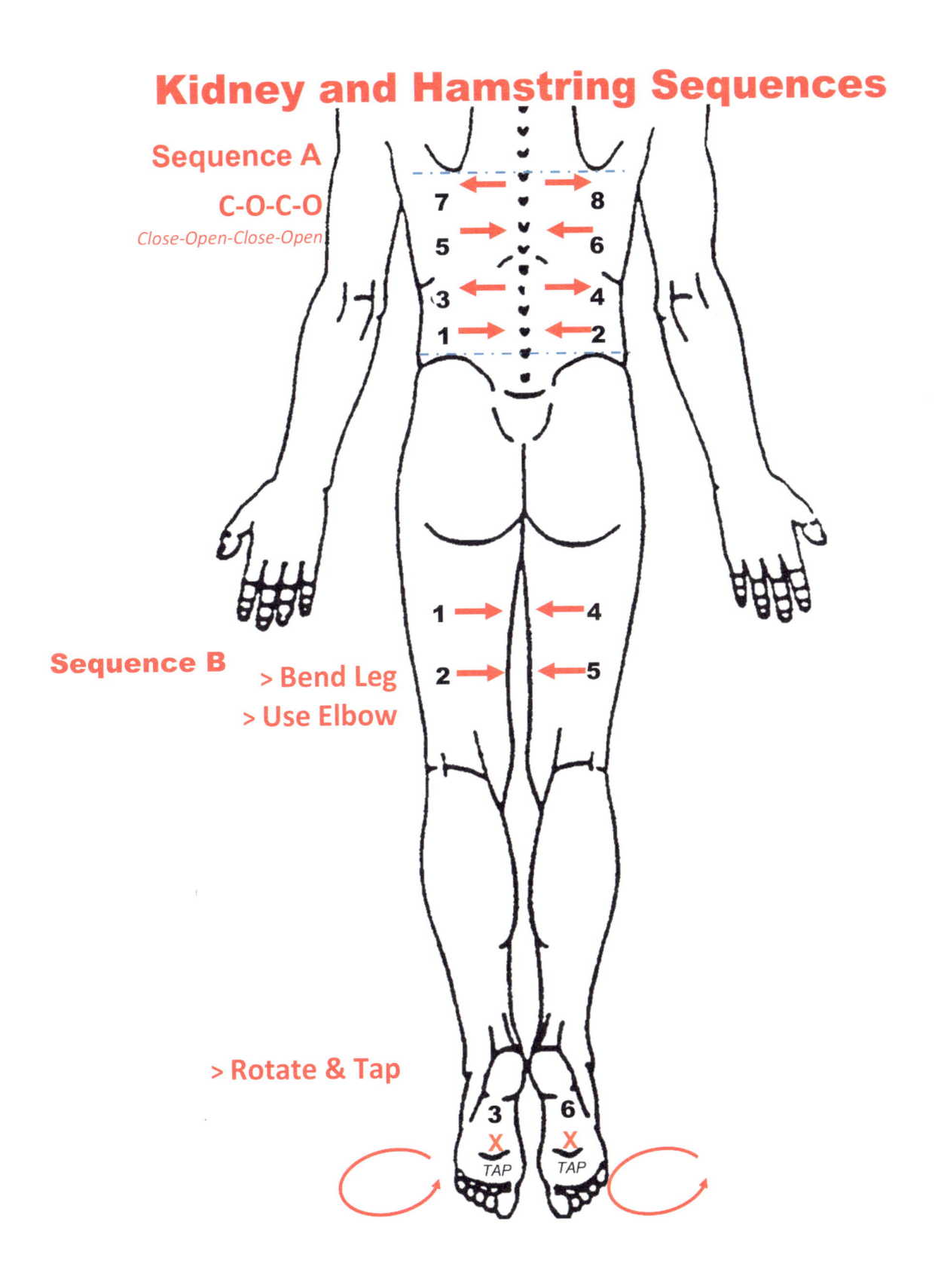

> Bend Leg
> Use Elbow

1 → ← 4
2 → ← 5

> Rotate & Tap

3 X TAP   6 X TAP

Pause and Rest

Kidney and Respiratory

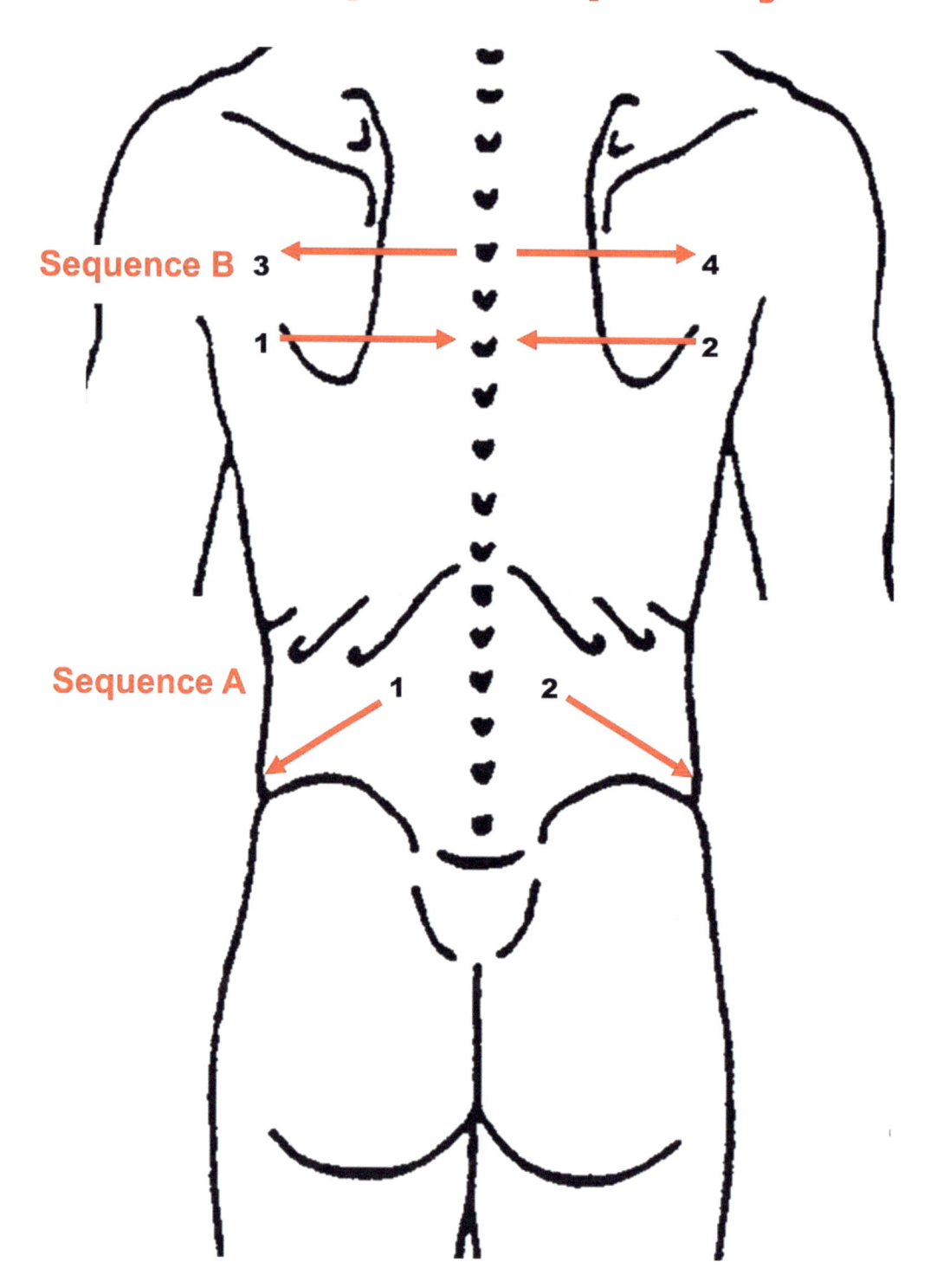

Sequence B 3 ← → 4

1 → ← 2

Sequence A 1 2

Pause and turn client over

Neck, Respiratory and Knee

Sequence A
Right SCM — 2
Left SCM — 1

Sequence B
Reach Behind to the Occipital
3 LEFT Rec. Cap. Major
4 RIGHT Rec. Cap. Major

Sequence C
Right / Left

Pause and Rest

Neck, Hamstring, Calf

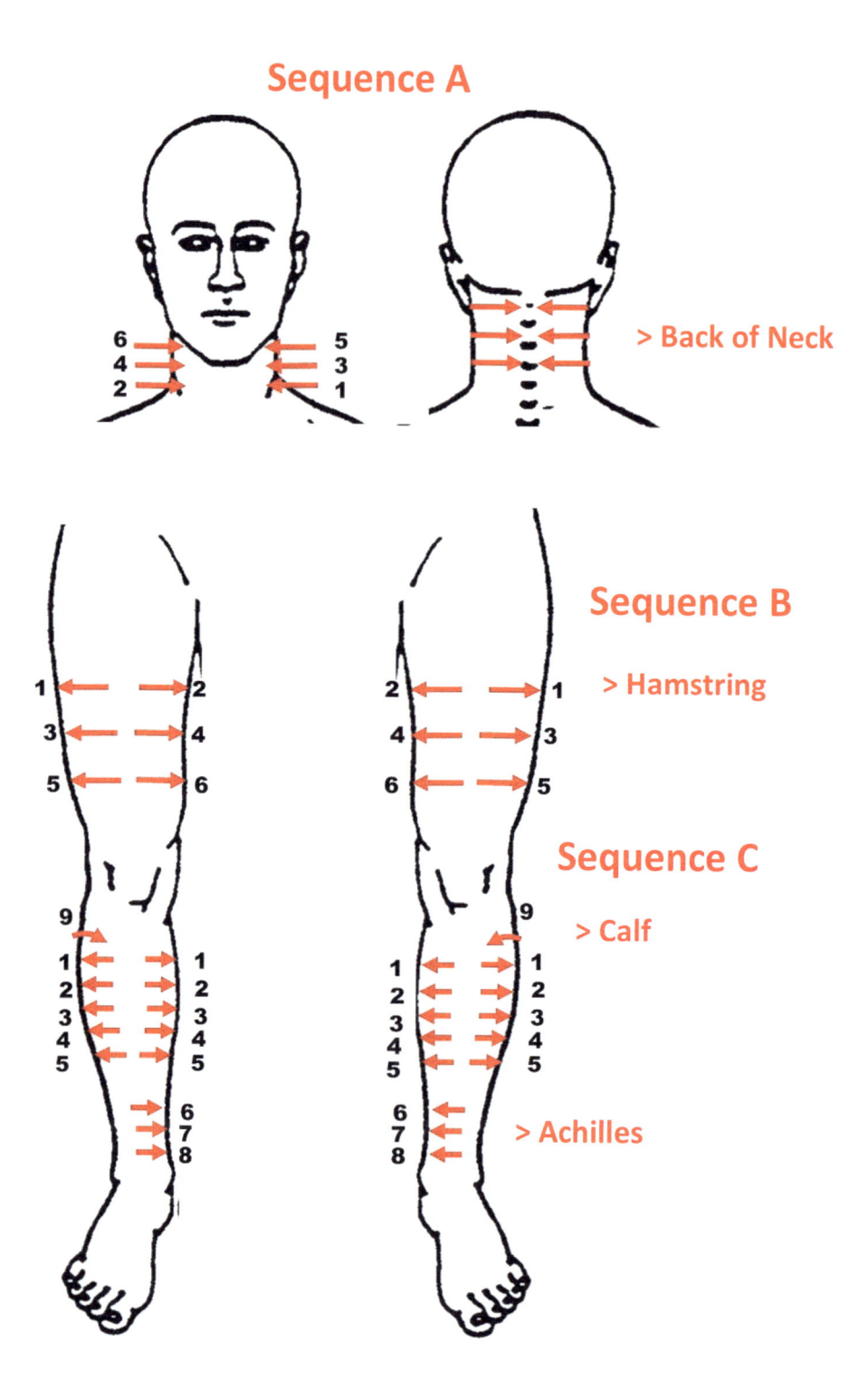

Sequence A

> Back of Neck

Sequence B

> Hamstring

Sequence C

> Calf

> Achilles

Pause and Rest

Copyright ©2018-2022 Michelle Lally, LMBT, Ca, NCBTMB, GA, FL | Ph: 704-929-9757 | www.BowsageTherapy.com

Knees, Pelvis & Upper Respiratory
Sequence A

1 → ← 1 < Calf
2 → ← 2
3 → ← 3
4 ↶ ↷ 4

Sequence B

4 → X   X ← 4
3 ↷   ↶ 3
2 ↶ ↷ 2
1 ↶   ↷ 1

> Itsy-Bitsy-Spider

Sequence C

10 ↓↓↓   9 ↓↓↓
2 ↘ ↙ 1
4↓ 3↓
6 → ← 5
8 → ← 7

Pause and Rest

Copyright ©2018-2022 Michelle Lally, LMBT, Ca, NCBTMB, GA, FL | Ph: 704-929-9757 | www.BowsageTherapy.com

TMJ, Breast & Ankle

Sequence A

Sequence B

Sequence C

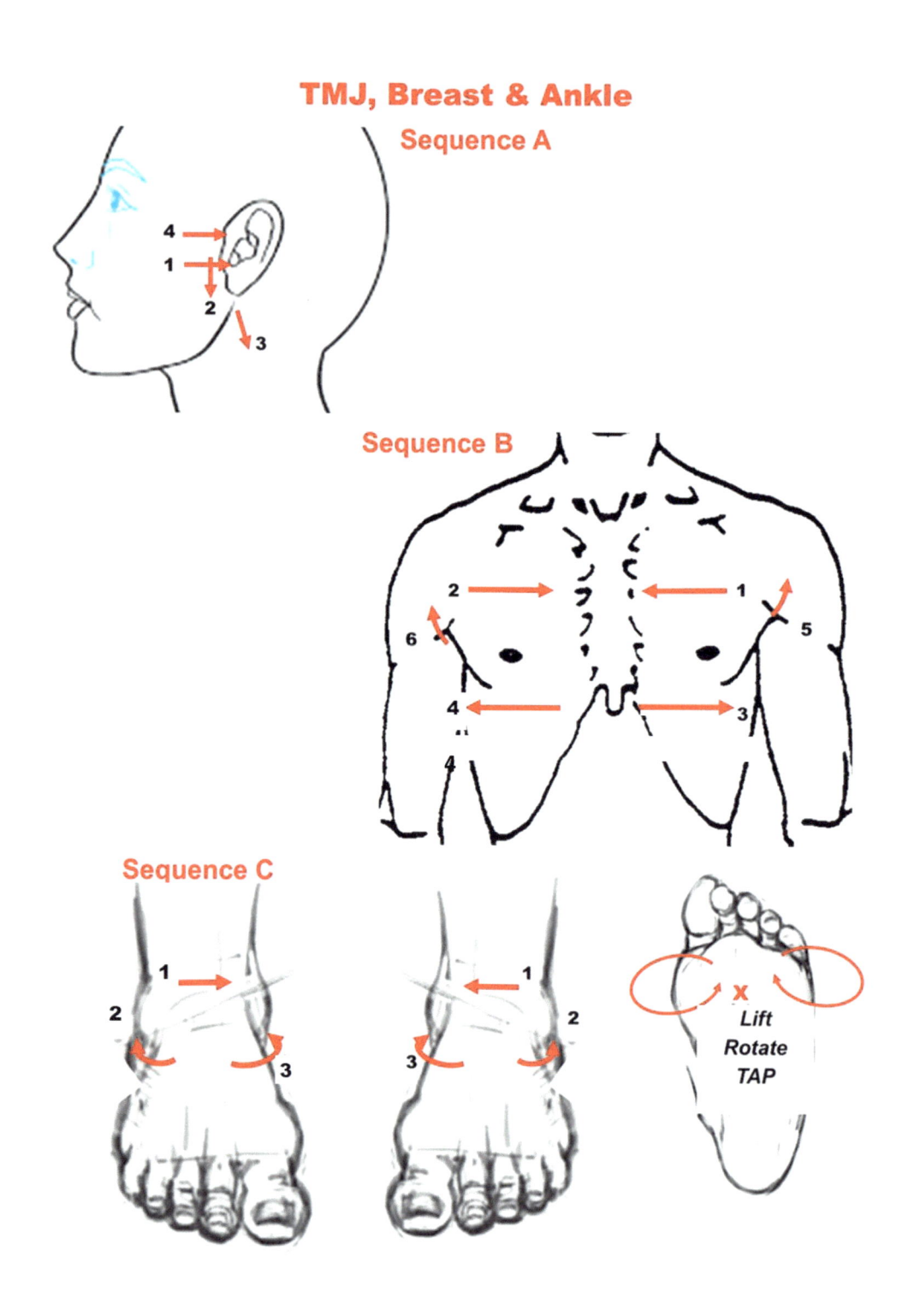

Lift
Rotate
TAP

Pause and Assist Client

Basic Relaxation 1 and 2

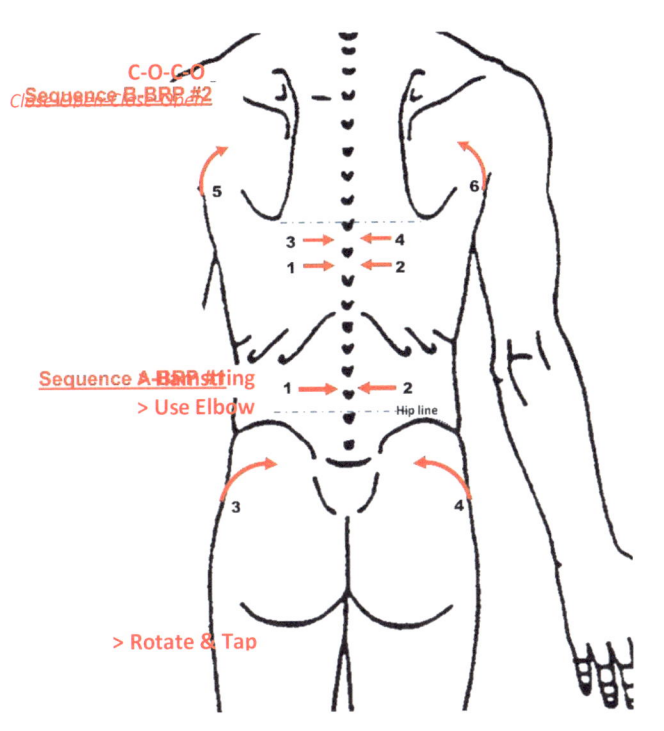

C-O-C-O
Sequence B-BRP #2
Closure B-BRP #2

Sequence A-BRP#1
Sequence A-Hamstring
> Use Elbow
Hip line

> Rotate & Tap

Basic Relaxation 3 and 4

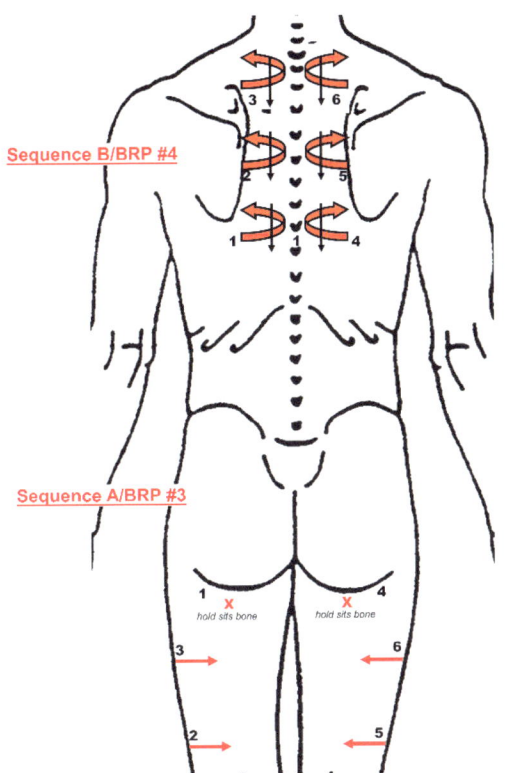

Sequence B/BRP #4

Sequence A/BRP #3

X hold sits bone   X hold sits bone

Kidney and Hamstring Sequences

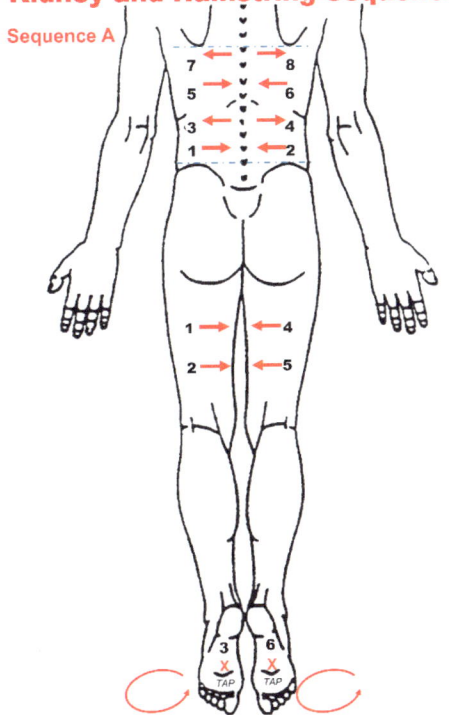

Sequence A

TAP   TAP

Kidney and Respiratory

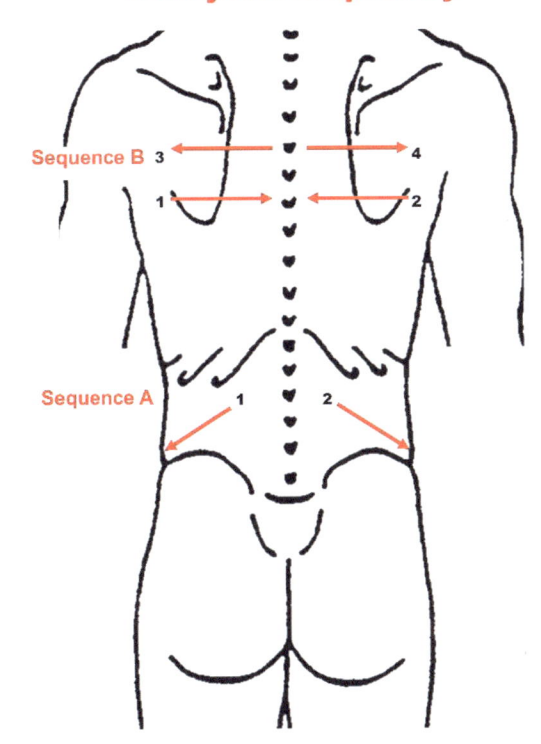

Sequence B

Sequence A

Neck, Respiratory and Knee

Sequence A

Right SCM / Left SCM

Reach Behind to the Occipital

LEFT — Rec. Cap. Major
RIGHT — Rec. Cap. Major

Sequence B

Right / Left

Sequence C

Neck, Hamstring, Calf

Sequence A

> Back of Neck

Sequence B

> Hamstring

Sequence C

> Calf

> Achilles

Knees, Pelvis & Upper Respiratory

Sequence A

< Calf

Sequence B — Itsy-Bitsy-Spider

Sequence C

TMJ, Breast & Ankle

Sequence A

Sequence B

Sequence C

X — Lift Rotate TAP

Copyright ©2018-2022 Michelle Lally, LMBT, Ca, NCBTMB, GA, FL | Ph: 704-929-9757 | www.BowsageTherapy.com

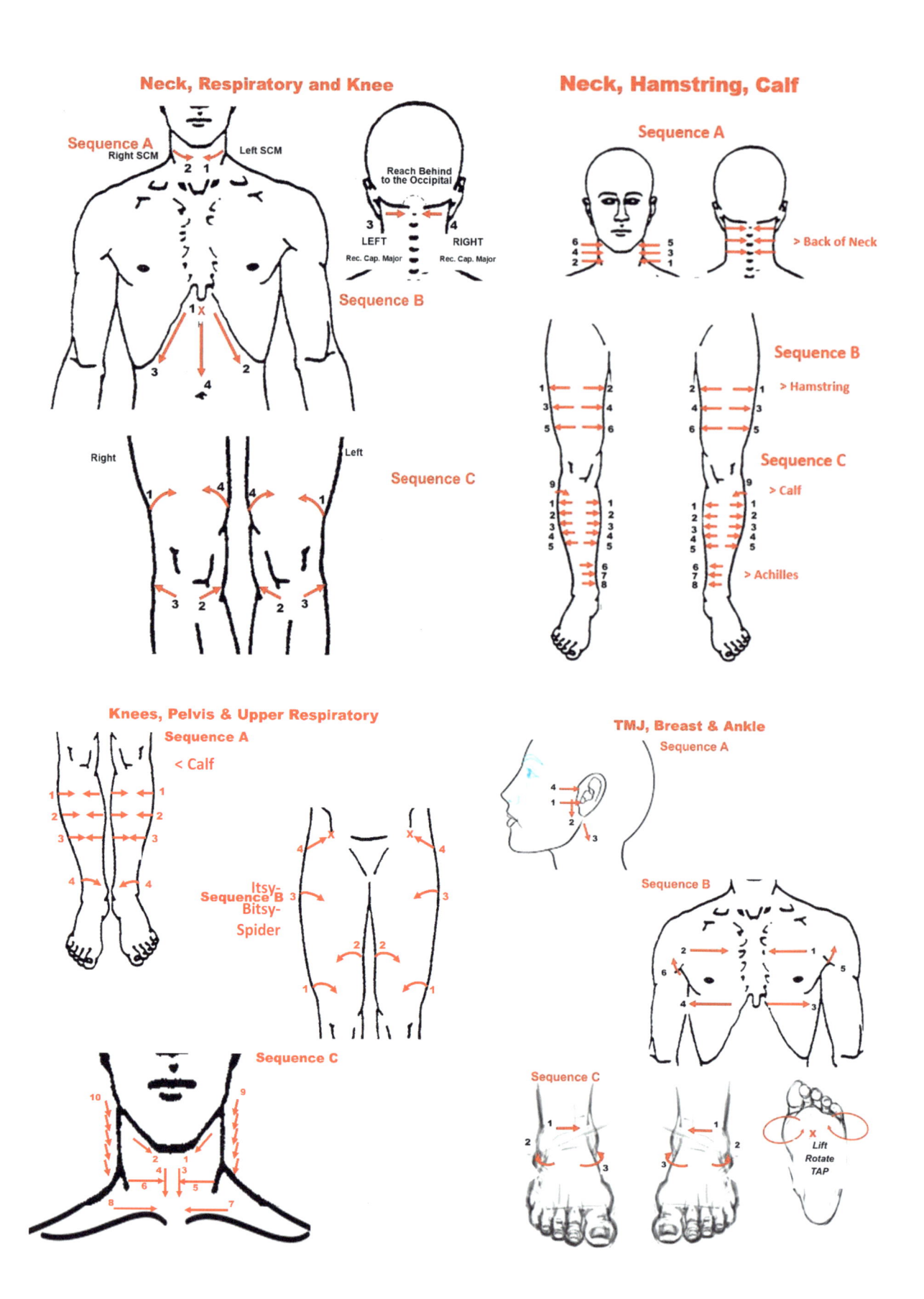

ARM PROCEDURE 1 / TENNIS ELBOW / CARPAL TUNNEL

Prerequisites: Basic relaxation procedures 1 – 2 – 3

Procedure: Client positioned on edge of table with legs hanging over. Do left side first unless injured, then do right first. Practitioner stands facing clients' left side.

1. Move 1: About 3 fingers below the top of the left shoulder in the middle of the deltoid muscle palpate for the head of the biceps [a clothesline like cord under the deltoid] using your right index finger. Remove slack posteriorly and begin slowly moving fingertips while increasing pressure as the muscle rolls under your fingertips to complete move 1.

2. Move 2: Hold clients' forearm in the webs between your thumbs pointing upward and your fingers pointed away. Move your right thumb over the extensor digitorum muscle in the upper anterior part of the forearm. Have client flex and extend the middle finger to confirm correct position, which can be palpated during contraction. Remove the skin slack toward the ulna and make a move over the muscle border toward the radius with your thumb. The clients' middle finger should twitch if done properly. This completes move 2.

3. Move 3: Cup the flexed left elbow in your left hand and place your fingertips above the lateral epicondyle of the humerus over the long head of the triceps. Remove slack posteriorly slowly increasing pressure and moving the muscle anterior to complete move 3.

4. Move 4: Holding points X – Y– Z: Place the fingers of your right hand behind the triceps over the humerus. Slide your index and middle fingers toward the elbow until they stop at the lateral and medial epicondyles of the humerus. Your index finger will rest at the lateral epicondyle [X]., and your middle finger will rest at the medial epicondyle [Y]. Next, place your thumb over the radial nerve where the radius and lateral epicondyles meet [Z]. Apply pressure to the 3 points for 10 seconds. The fingers will become numb for a moment. Then release pressure.

5. Move 5: Grasp clients' wrist with both hands keeping the palm of the hand downward. Your right thumbs in the middle of the wrist remove slack laterally and move medially over the tendons.

6. Move 6: Open the wrist by grasping the wrist with both hands A. your left thumb anterior to the radius. B. Your right thumb anterior to the ulna. C. & D. Place your index and middle fingers on the opposite side of the wrist from your thumbs. By randomly moving the wrist up and down and back and forth while applying a little traction the wrist will open. Many times, a little click will be palpable or audible.

7. Move 7: These are double moves to open the forearm the same as when the hamstrings are opened. Remove slack medially and move the muscle laterally. Then repeat on the other side by removing slack lateral and make the move medially. Move down the forearm an inch and repeat. Continue down the arm until you reach the wrist.

8. Move 8: Close the forearm muscles by gently squeezing the muscles together beginning at the top of the forearm and ending at the wrist.

ARM PROCEDURE 1

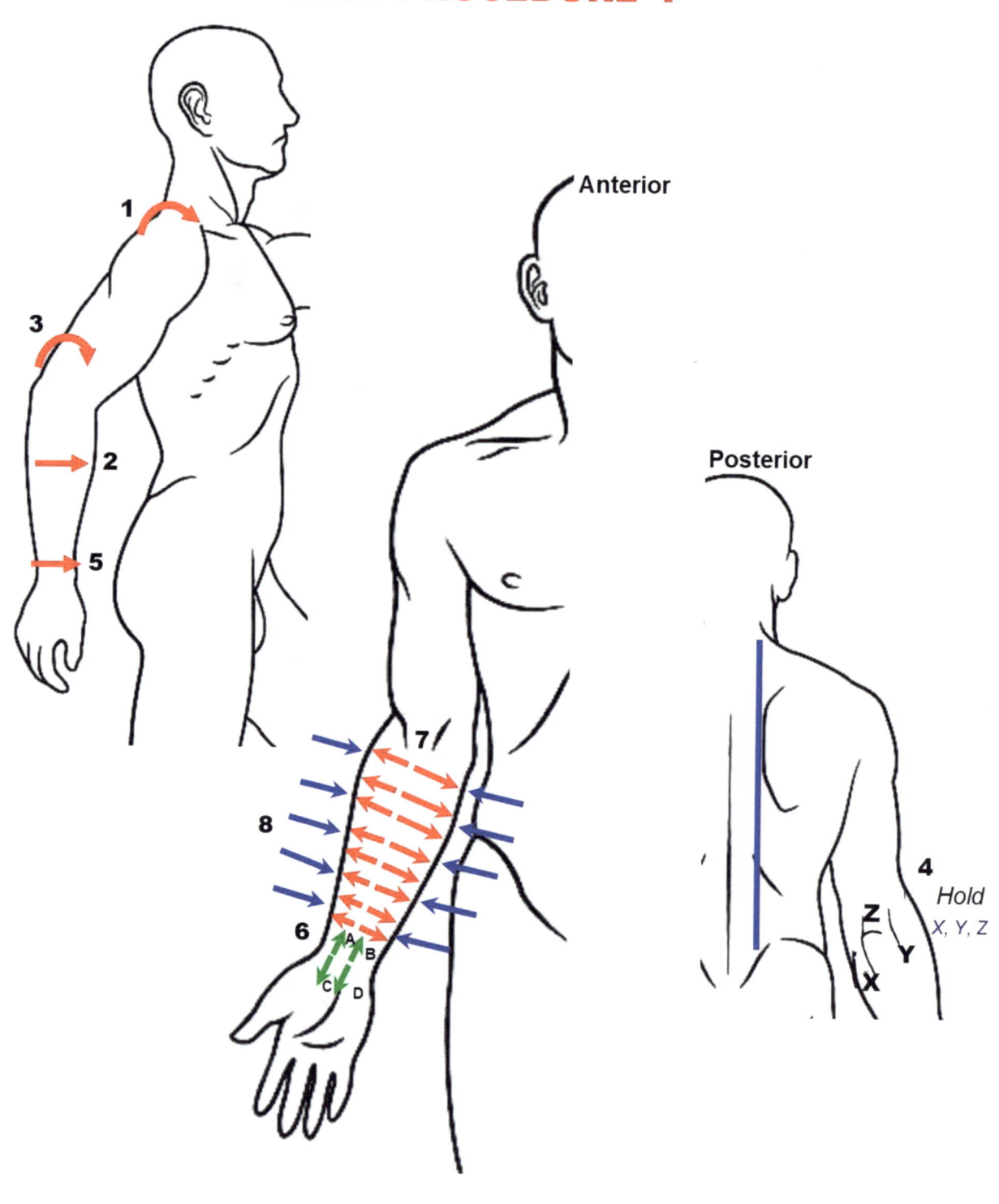

Anterior

Posterior

Hold X, Y, Z

ARM PROCEDURE 2

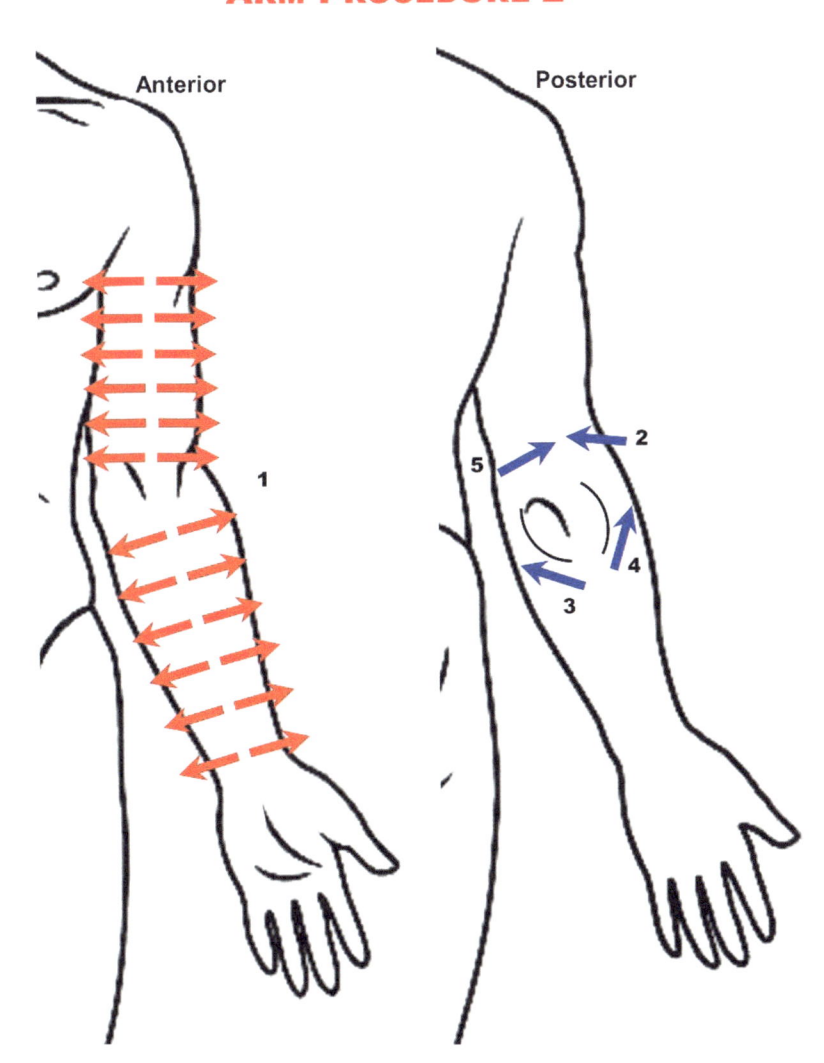

Client in supine or sitting position.

Prerequisites: Basic Relaxation Procedures 2 & 3, Shoulder 1 & Arm 1

Procedure: Red arrows = random separation of upper arm and forearm muscles.

1. Slide both hands up inside arm into the axillary fold. Using your fingertips move the upper arm muscles lateral and medial about 1 inch apart down to the elbow. Continue these moves from elbow to wrist.

2. Moves 2-3-4-5: are the same moves as the knee procedure.

SHOULDER PROCEDURE AKA FROZEN SHOULDER

Always do the less painful side first. If neither side painful, do the left side first.

Prerequisites: Basic relaxation procedures 1 – 2 – 3.

Procedure: Client sits on the edge of the table facing the practitioner with legs hanging over the edge of the table. Practitioner stands on clients' right side facing the left shoulder. Place your right knee between clients' legs. Bend the clients' left elbow 90 degrees and cradle the elbow in your left hand. Let clients' forearm rest on your forearm.

1. Move 1: Place your right thumb under the posterior border of the deltoid muscle just above the axilla. Remove slack inferiorly and apply pressure as client takes in a deep breath. On the exhale, begin moving the elbow toward the right shoulder in your left hand as your right thumb rolls over the edge of the deltoid. If the proper release is obtained you will feel a vibration in the insertion of the triceps at the medial epicondyle of the humerus in your left hand under your thumb. If there is no response, repeat the move. Maintain the fully adducted shoulder position and firmly strike the lateral aspect of the shoulder with the heel of your right hand. Gently return the clients' shoulder to neutral to complete move 1.

2. Move 2: Place your right thumb below the anterior border of the deltoid muscle. Remove slack inferiorly and move the muscle border superiorly to complete move 2.

3. Repeat moves 1 & 2 if needed.

4. Move toward clients' left side; place your left knee between client's legs, and repeat moves on the right shoulder.

(DIAGRAM NEXT PAGE)

Shoulder Procedure 1

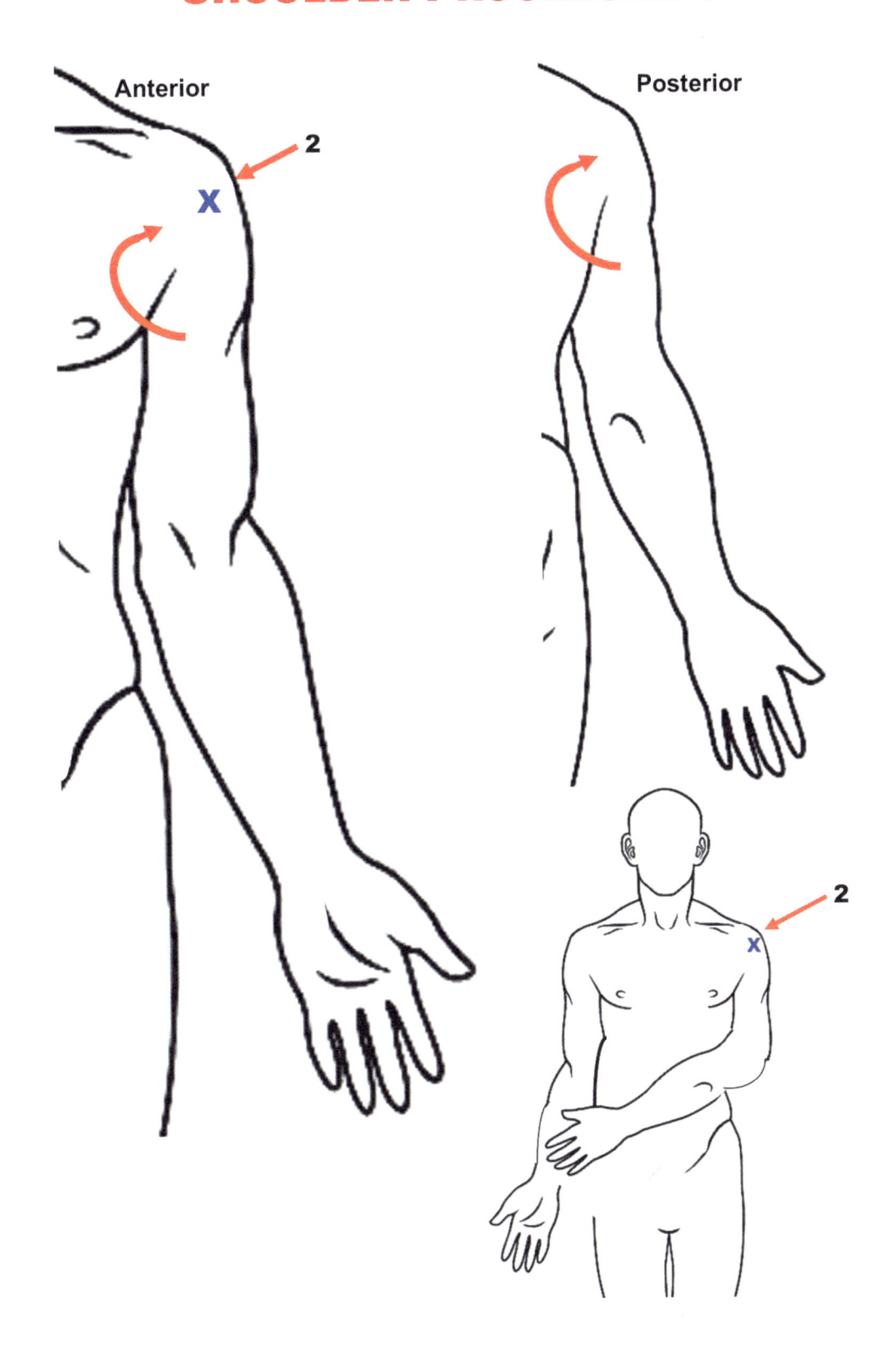

Anterior

Posterior

2

CERVICAL RELEASE

This technique is a combination of craniosacral and fascial release procedures. Within the craniosacral system there's a rhythm, as there's a heart rhythm, and there's a respiratory rhythm. This rhythm can be palpated by the practitioner at a number of different points with a little bit of practice and patience.

Procedure: Client supine. Practitioner seated at the head of the table. Place your cupped hands beneath the client's head with the tips of your fingers just beneath the base of the skull. Tell your client that you are going to wait for them to relax a minute.

1. Gently stretch their neck straight [cephalad], toward the right, then toward the left, and then back to neutral.

2. Feel for the expansion of your hands as the cranial bones expand, pause, and then contract.

3. After a minute you will be able to perceive these fluctuations to the rate of 6 to 10 per minute. On one of the inward contractions maintain gentle resistance to the outward expansion phase. Continue to hold in this manner until you feel a tapping-thumping-fluttering under your palms.

    a. Breathing may change, the stomach may gurgle, toes may wiggle, beads of perspiration may appear, and skin color may change. When the sensations become quiet under your palms the client has reached a "Still point", which is therapeutic in and by itself.

    b. Maintain steady gentle superior traction and mentally visualize the dura tube stretching inside the spinal canal while you silently count down; "Atlas-axis-C3-C4-C5-C6-C7-T1-T2-T3-T4-T5-T6-T7-T8-T9-T10-T11-T12-L1-L2-L3-L4-L5-S1-S2-S3-S4-S5-COCCYX1-COCCYX 2".

4. While maintaining the gentle steady traction, begin turning the head very slowly to the right and repeat the count down and visualization procedure, which will stretch the left side of the dura fascia.

5. When completed, slowly begin moving the head to the left and complete the stretch on the right side of the dura fascia in the same fashion.

6. When complete, return head to neutral, hold and wait for the rhythm to return. Return of the rhythm may take seconds to a minute or 2. The rhythm may begin at a very shallow rate and gradually become fuller. At this time you may welcome your client back to reality.

7. This technique helps to remove sympathetic overloading, brings on parasympathetic "Rest and digest", and may help to reduce spinal nerve irritations and anomalies. Very often hands and feet will warm both temporarily, and sometimes permanently. A variation of this technique has been documented to reduce fever by 3 to 5 degrees.

Once you perform this for a client, you'll rarely be able to dismiss them from a session until you repeat it.

THE CHAIR-SIDE RE-BOOT

Based on feedback I received over the years, I put together a 5-minute chair-side Bowen Session, which includes 2-minute rests. I call it, "The Chair-side Re-Boot". Feedback has been positive and can be offered as a $10 session. Clients should be encouraged to get a session once a week for 3 weeks. It works on:

- Muscle tension and stress release
- Headaches
- Neck problems
- Shoulder problems
- Carpal tunnel & Tennis elbow
- Low back & Hip pain

Applications are:
- As a demonstration
- As a free introductory session
- To work in a last-minute emergency request
- As a part of the full routine session
- For a quick tune up
- For workplace settings for occupational enhancement

CHAIRSIDE RE-BOOT PROCEDURE

Prerequisites: None

Procedure: Position the client comfortably on a massage chair or standing (optional position).

Part A.*
1. BRP 1 A
2. BRP 2 A
3. BRP 3 A
REST   1 – 2 minutes.

Part B.
1. BRP 1 B
2. BRP 2 B
3. BRP 3 B
REST 1 – 2 minutes

Part C.
1. 10 compressions @ Cranial Base with middle finger.

DEEP RELAXATION (OPTIONAL) PROCEDURE

Use this when your client is in so much pain that they can't get up on the table. It will relax them so they can move a little better prior to getting up on the table. I found this procedure helpful for patients who were in acute spasms and could not climb up. It enabled them to be slightly more mobile, and it only took a minute or so to do.

Procedure: Client stands facing you with their hands on your shoulders. Reach behind with both hands and place your fingertips just above the crest of the ilium over the middle of the erector spinae muscles.

1. With your right-hand push slack medially and hold pressure against the muscle for 3 seconds. As you increase the pressure straighten your fingertips, so the muscle rolls out from under your fingertips. The move is made 30 degrees superiorly and laterally.
2. Repeat with your left hand on the client's right side.
3. Move your hands up the spine 2 inches on the left and repeat the process.
4. Repeat the same on the right.
5. Move up another 2 inches and repeat left.
6. Repeat right.
7. Add additional oblique moves until you reach the mid scapula region. If there is any tenderness along the way up have client take deep breaths between repeat moves. You may repeat the sequence 3 time if needed.
8. Reposition your hands so your middle fingers are resting on the coccyx hold point [sacral notch]. Move slack inferior toward the coccyx with your right hand, and then make an oblique move 45 degrees superior and laterally over the reflex point to complete move
9. Repeat with your left hand on the right side. Have client breath in and out deeply and take a few steps.
10. Repeat 8 & 9 if still tender.

This procedure is highly effective by itself as a warm-up, or if a client has difficulty laying prone on the table, do this procedure to loosen them up first. It may also be used if your client experiences any kidney / low back discomfort following a regular session. Also, if time and space does not allow for a full session at the time, this can be done in a hallway or waiting room in your office.

(DIAGRAM NEXT PAGE)

Deep Relaxation Procedure (optional)

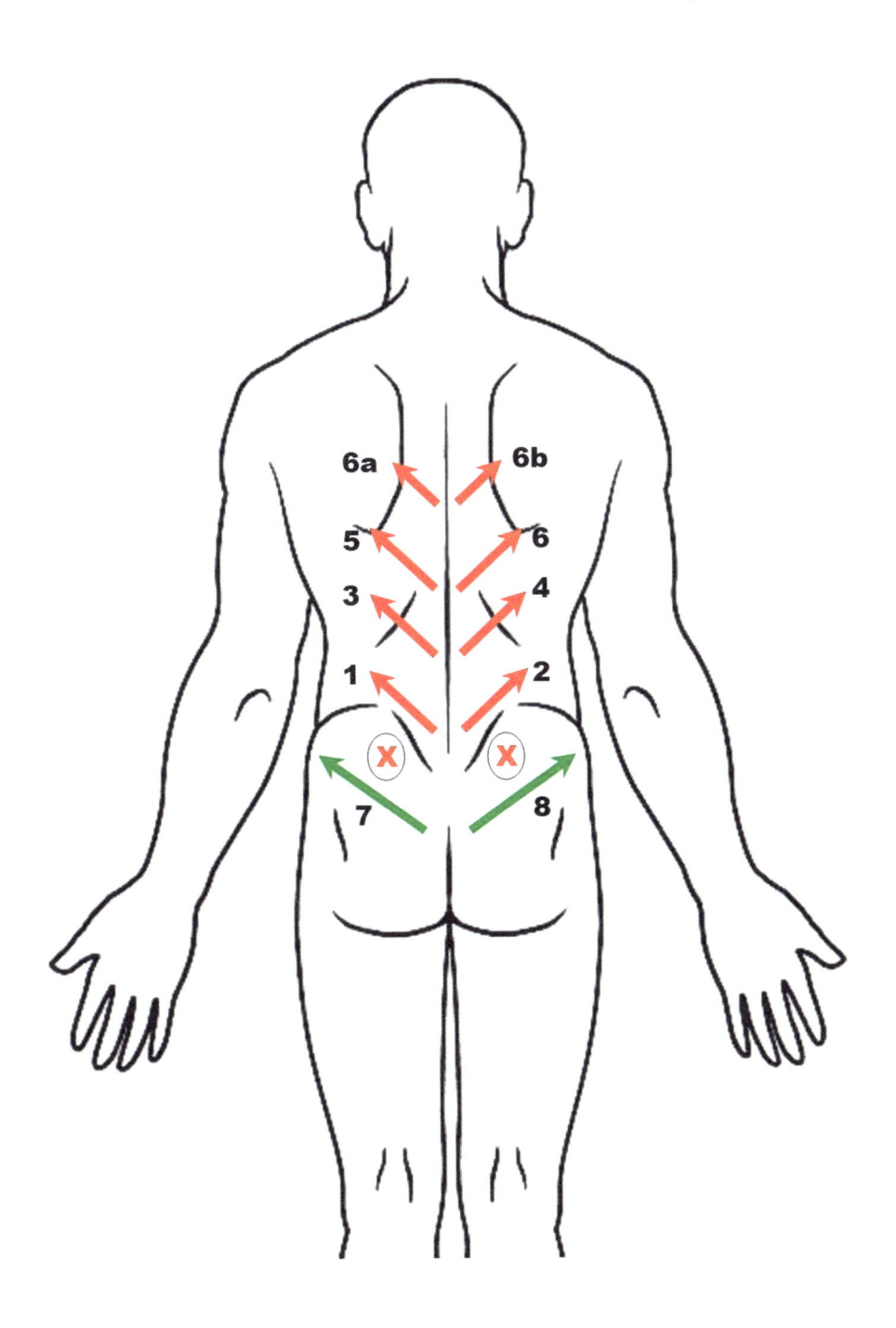

COCCYX PROCEDURE

Prerequisites: Basic relaxation procedure moves 1 through 4 **Caution**: *Do not do the coccyx move on pregnant women. Do not do both sides. Do not repeat on the same visit. Part B move can be beneficial to clients with IBS, and infants with colic.*

Part A. Client in prone position.

1. Turn the head toward the left shoulder and tuck the chin.

2. Place your middle finger of the left hand on the top of the coccyx bone and follow it down to the tip of the coccyx. Feel for any deviations to the right, left, or anterior. Press lightly on the left mid part of the coccyx and determine any tenderness.

3. Repeat light pressure on the right side of the coccyx. If the right side is tender the move is on the right side. If neither side is tender, nor the left side is tender, then the move is on the left side.

4. Practitioner stands on the side of the client upon which side is to receive the move. Return the head toward the same side and tuck the chin toward the shoulder. Doing the left side, grasp the left leg with your right hand, place your middle finger on the posterior tibial nerve behind the internal [medial] malleolus, bend the leg at the knee to 90 deg.

5. Place your thumb over the peroneal retinaculum beneath the lateral malleolus and rotate the leg laterally until the leg engages the trunk.

6. Apply slight pressure to reflex point 1 with your 3rd finger and relocate your index finger on the lateral border of the coccyx midway, point 2.

7. Remove slack laterally with your index finger while maintaining slight pressure on the reflex point 1 during client's inhale.

8. Move your index finger medially with light pressure on the client's exhale. Return leg to 90 deg. Then back to the table.

9. Rest period 5 minutes- then turn client to the supine position.

Part B. Client in supine position:

1. If the move was on the left side, practitioner stands on client's left side.

2. Move the leg laterally 6 inches using your left hand.

3. Then flex the knee by holding your left hand below the knee.

4. Place your index and middle fingers of your right hand ½ way between the umbilicus and the inguinal ligament, point 3.

5. Begin moving the leg and knee toward the right shoulder and have client take a deep breath as the knee becomes flexed to 90 deg.

6. Continue moving the knee toward the shoulder on the exhale and move your fingers at the same time toward the umbilicus to remove the slack, then rotate your hand and move toward the left ribs.

7. Gently straighten the leg and return it to the table center. This locks the coccyx.

Part C. Client in supine position:

1. Have the client raise the left leg straight upward as high as it will go, then flex the knee, lowering the foot toward the table and at the ½ way point extend the knee. Then lower the straightened leg back to the tabletop.

2. Have client drag the left foot back along the tabletop until the knee is flexed maximally, then raise leg until extended straight. Raise leg upward as high as it will go, pause and then slowly lower back to the tabletop. This same move is used to lock the pelvis after the anterior pelvis moves.

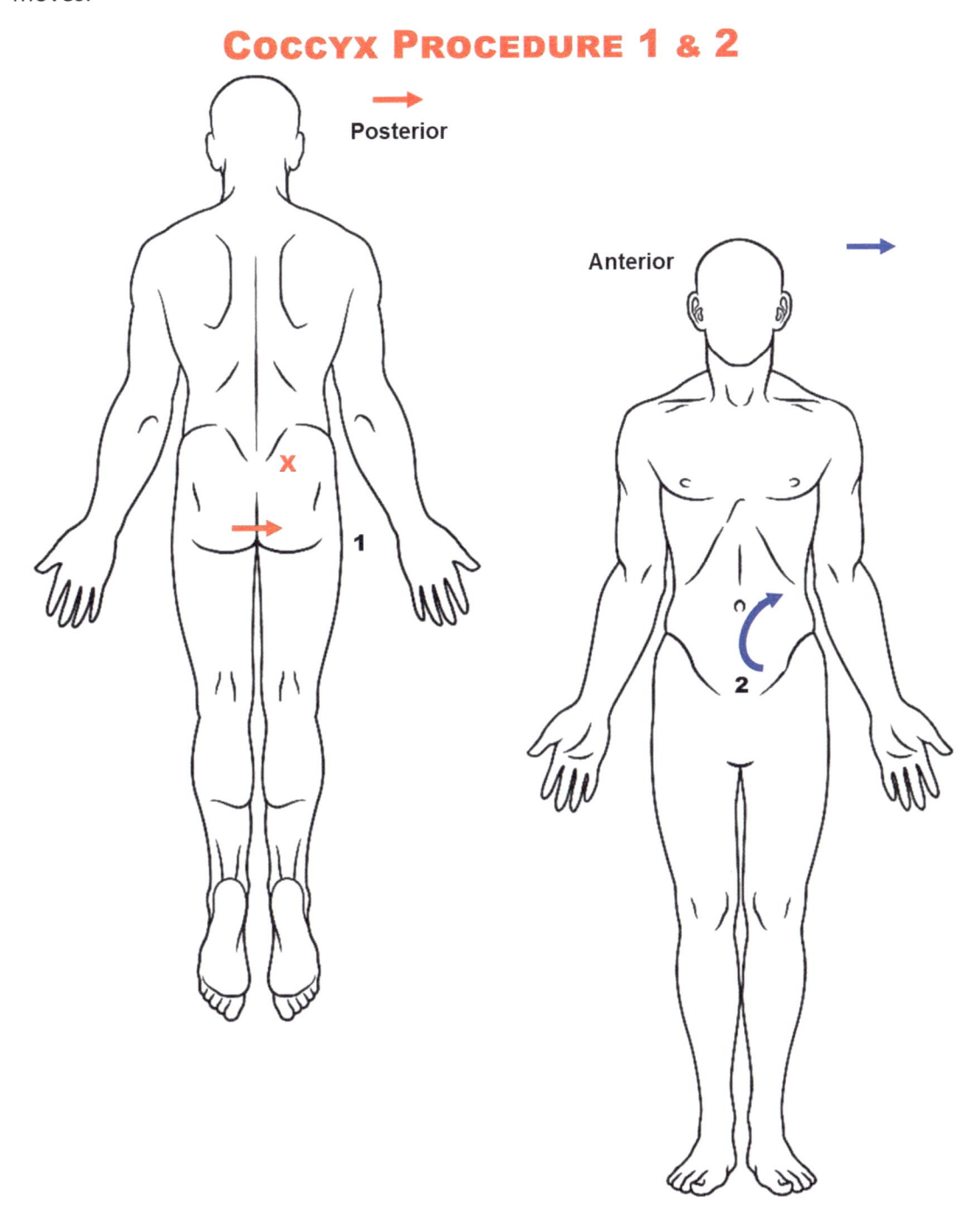

COCCYX PROCEDURE 1 & 2

DIAPHRAGM RELEASES

There are 6 transverse diaphragms. They are: 1) pelvis floor, 2) respiratory diaphragm, 3) thoracic inlet/outlet, 4) hyoid, 5) cranial base, and 6) joint capsules [synovial membranes are also considered transverse diaphragms].

When these fibro-muscular tissues become distorted there is a deforming force exerted on their attachments. The structures that pass through the diaphragms, [nerves, blood & lymph vessels, meridian channels, and other electrical conduits] can be mildly compressed and rendered dysfunctional. Positional postural changes [pelvic & shoulder tilts], intrauterine & intra-abdominal pressure, traumatic events including surgeries may all have a role in the distortion process. Keep in mind that the crus ligaments attach the posterior respiratory diaphragm to L4 –L5, pressure exerted in an upward direction against the diaphragm will place tension on these ligaments and cause low back pain.

You do not have to perform releases at every diaphragm. For instance, with low back pain do the pelvic and respiratory. For carpal tunnel or arm pain do the thoracic and hyoid. We usually do these following the completed Bowen session; however, you can do them at the beginning of the session if you feel that is warranted for this client.

Procedure: To release the *pelvis*:

1. Place one hand behind the sacrum and the other over the lower abdominal area.
2. In order to place the heel of your hand just above the pubis, slowly slide down while pressing downward into the tissue until your hand rests on the top of the pubis.
3. Also, have your client locate the top of the pubic bone with their first 2 fingers then place the heel of your hand just above.
4. Lightly engage the tissue with your upper hand fingers pointing laterally.
5. Wait for a slight indication of movement in one direction or another and go with it. Allow your hand to move with the tissue movement. Do not be surprised at anything. If there is no movement after a minute or two move on to the respiratory diaphragm.

To release the *respiratory diaphragm*:

1. Place one hand behind the area of T -12.
2. Place the palm of your upper hand beneath the xiphoid process with fingers pointing toward the head. Lightly engage the tissue and wait for a response and subsequent movement. Follow the movement wherever it goes, and for how long it takes to unwind to a still point. If there is no movement in a minute or two move up to the thoracic Diaphragm.

To release the ***thoracic diaphragm***:

1. Place one hand behind the thoracic spine between the scapula on both sides and the other on top of the clavicle, [thumb pointing toward you on one clavicle and your index finger pointing away from you on the opposite clavicle].

2. Lightly engage the tissue and wait for a response and subsequent movement. Follow the steps outlined above.

To release the ***hyoid diaphragm***:

1. Place one hand behind the neck and with the other hand place your fingers together and spread your thumb – like you are going to hold a glass in your hand.

2. Gently place your hand –fingers on one side and thumb on the other side just above the thyroid cartilage and under the mandibles. Follow the steps outlined above.

To release the ***cranial base diaphragm***

1. Lift the head upward with both hands cupped.

2. Place the fingertips of the cupped hand into the soft tissue at the base of the skull and then balance the cranium on your fingertips only.

3. If the cranium rocks back and forth, maintain the balance point until it stabilizes.

4. Within a minute or two the cranium will usually drop down into the palm of your hands. When this occurs use your intent and imagine the dural tube inside the vertebral canal elongating as you count down the vertebral spine in your thought. When you reach C3 at the coccyx you are finished.

DIAPHRAGM PROCEDURE

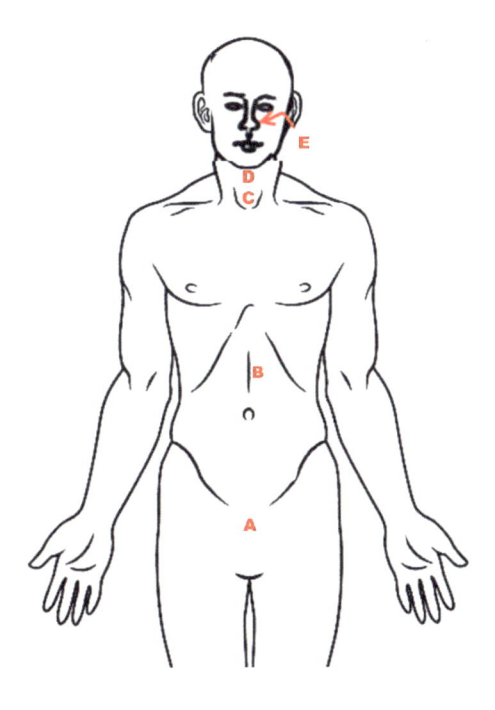

DIGESTIVE - ABDOMINAL PROCEDURE

Use for any digestive and or abdominal complaints.

Prerequisites: Basic Relaxation procedures 1 and 2, Respiratory Procedure & Torso Procedure

Procedure: Client in prone position. Wait 2 minutes.

1. Moves 1 & 2: Lateral moves over the vagus nerve.
2. Moves 3 & 4: Cross shaped moves above pubis over the pubic nerves.
3. Moves 5 & 6: Clockwise circles ending with a superior-medial move toward the umbilicus. Use 3 fingers and medium pressure.
4. Move 5 stimulates the sigmoid flexure.
5. Move 6 stimulates the ileocecal valve
6. Moves 7-8-9: Use 3 middle fingers with medium pressure toward umbilicus.

Note: Moves 5-9 are in a clockwise direction. Lower left to upper left.

QUICK PROCEDURES

For baby with colic: Have mom hold and do coccyx lock [part B] on both sides plus Kidney Procedure.

For adult with IBS-diarrhea-cramps in stomach: Do coccyx lock [part B] both sides

(DIAGRAM NEXT PAGE)

Abdominal Procedure

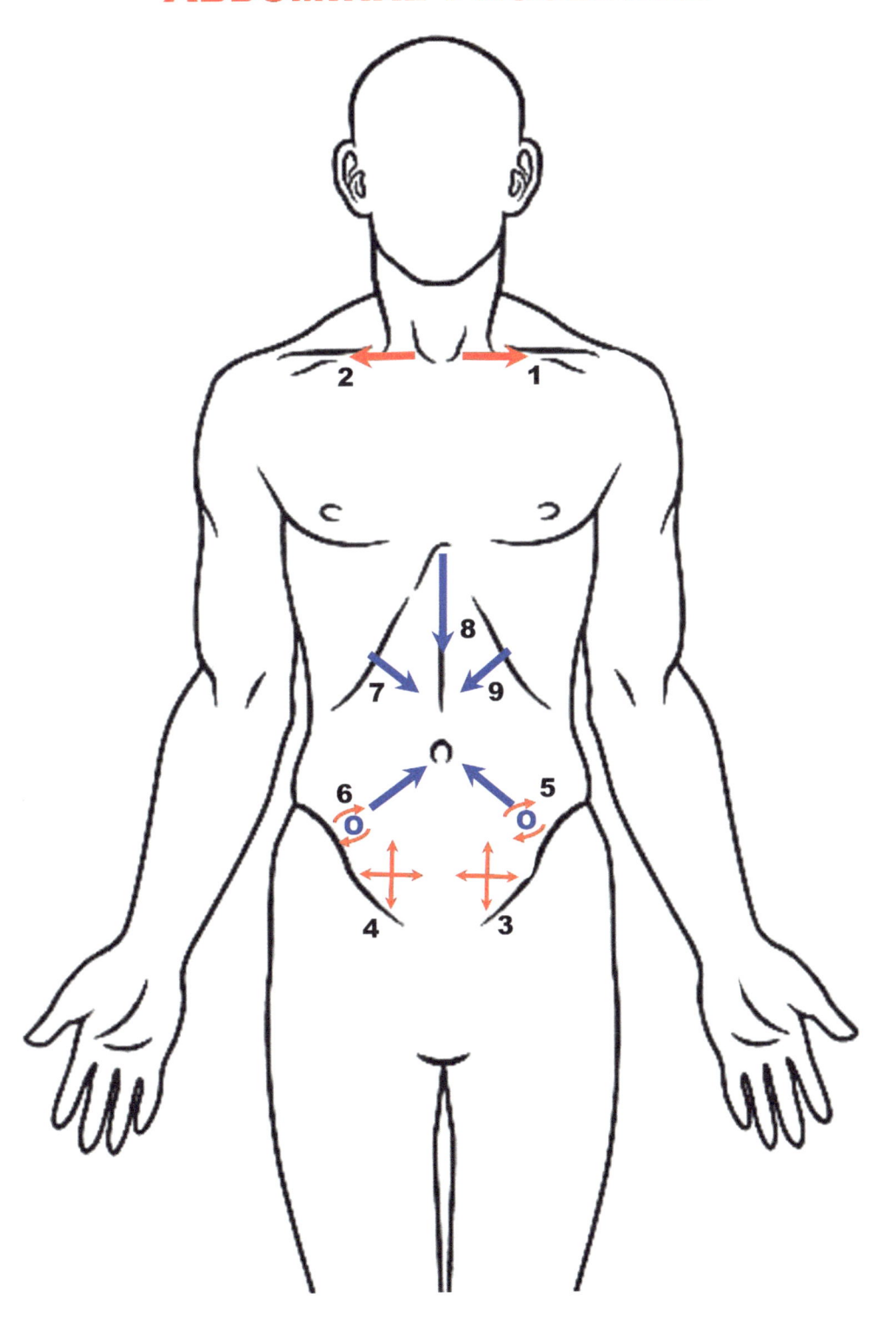

TORSO PROCEDURE

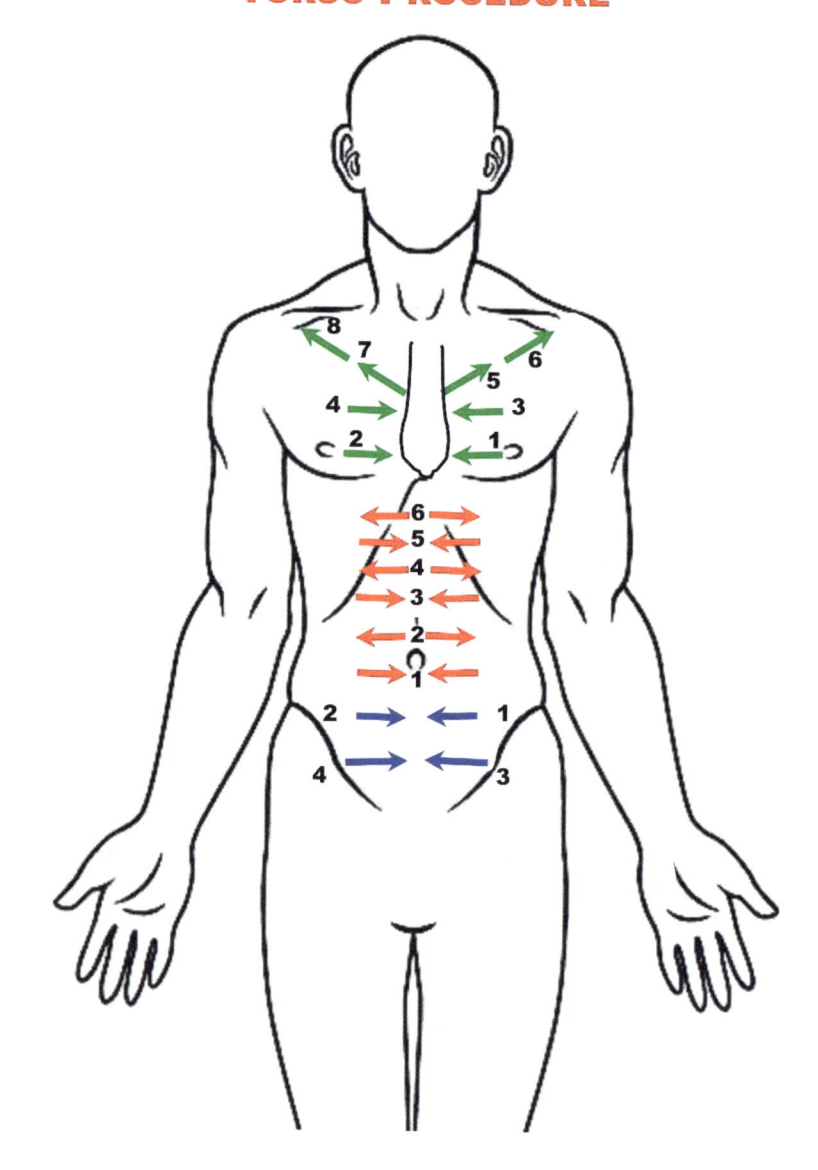

Prerequisites: Basic Relaxation Procedures 1-2-3, Kidney – Respiratory, Vastus lateralis, Hay Fever & TMJ

Procedure: Wait 2 minutes

1. Do moves 1 – 4 blue arrows, Wait 2 minutes
2. Do moves 1 – 8 green arrows, Wait 2 minutes
3. Do moves 1 – 6 red arrows [each number has 2 moves]

Note: 1 – 3 – 5 are medial moves, 2 – 4 – 6 are lateral moves

EMOTIONAL CLEARING PROCEDURE

The case history below illustrates the power of the body-mind connection. In other words, how to Ctrl-Alt-Delete, and how the subconscious mind can be influenced by something in writing connected with a body part. Masaru Emoto, a Japanese businessman and author who claimed that human speech or thoughts have dramatic effects on water, proved that water crystals can be influenced by the written word, spoken word, thought, music, and picture. Since humans are comprised of about 60% water, you can see how words can affect the water cells in our bodies.

Client case: I had referred Jan to a naturopath friend for allergy clearings who referred her back to me. Apparently, she was holding on to some symptoms due to holding on to an emotion which was blocking the clearing process. My friend called and asked me if Bowen could help her by inducing an emotional release. I said, "It might. I have had a number of patients release spontaneously over the years, so I could give it a try". This was prior to my learning about emotional release from John Barnes and John Upledger.

In the first session we both intended that she release whatever negative emotion she would like to release at that time. Nothing happened. We attempted this approach a second time, with a little more intent, at least on my part. Still no response. We proceeded with a third session and this time I asked her what the issue was she was trying to release. She told me the details about an incident with her father at age 5, who made her very angry, and she had never forgiven him for it. I asked her to write the following on a piece of paper, "I release all of my anger toward my father because of what he did to me." She held this in her left hand during a full body Basic Bowen session. That's all. Since then, I think that it is more effective to hold the paper in the right hand. The right hand is our giving hand, and what we want to do is to give away the emotional baggage we want to release.

She returned a week later to report that she had experienced a great deal of anger toward her children for two days following the session. But then it had disappeared along with the physical symptoms she had been dealing with the past years. I heard from her two years later and she had re-married, was living a calm and peaceful life without any anger issues or other physical ones.

Her success inspired the idea to clear other body-mind dysfunctions which can lead to cravings, allergies, weight gain or other unwanted health issues.

Prerequisites: None

Procedure: Client in a prone position for Basic Bowen Reset

Begin to discuss the possibility of some emotion that they felt they are hanging onto.

Once they identify the emotion or emotional situation, they can write it on a piece of paper in a similar fashion as this example: "I release all of my anger toward (person name here) because of what that person said or did to me."

Have them hold it in their left (confusing here as he indicated earlier that the right hand is better for releasing) [Emotional stuff in the right hand], hand during their regular Bowen Reset session. It is not important that you know what they wrote. Sometimes the release takes place during the session. Other times, they may feel the release later that day or over the next few days.

HAMMERTOES

There are variances in, and many causes of hammertoes. A good rule of thumb is, that if the toe / toes are flexible, there is a chance they may straighten with the proper release and rebalancing techniques. Remembering that there are many causative factors; elongated bones causing retrograde shoe and stocking pressure with buckling of the joints, weakened interossei and lumbricales muscles from low back denervation, prolonged use of high heel shoes which deviates the axis of the M-P joints and weakens the lumbricales and interossei, post fracture of phalanges and metatarsals, repetitive M-P joint trauma [2nd most often], and idiopathic tightening of the long extensors, and or flexors, are the most common causes of hammertoes. When the boney structure is abnormal, or the joints are fused or dislocated, body Re-Set likely will not correct the deformities.

If your clients are having hammertoe surgery performed; it is a good idea to do a session about 2 to 3 days pre-op, follow with another 4 to 5 days post-op, and then once a week X 2. This will accelerate the healing process, reduce muscle spasms, and help to prevent reoccurrence of the deformity. This is a great rule to follow when your clients are going to have *any* surgery performed.

Prerequisite: BRP 1, Anterior and Posterior Pelvis, Knee, Hamstrings, Peroneals, Posterior and Anterior Tibial, and Ankle immediately before the Hammertoe moves 1 through 15.

Procedure: Client is in the supine position. Left side first, immediately following the Ankle procedure.

1. Make 4 *anterior* moves [slack lateral], over the extensor digitorum longus muscle [anterior-lateral lower leg] beginning superior and working distal toward the ankle.

2. Palpate the vibratory action with your finger resting on the tendon just proximal to the M-P Joint. The superior muscle fibers = 2nd toe, most inferior muscle fibers = 5th, 3rd and 4th are in between.

HAMMERTOES PROCEDURE

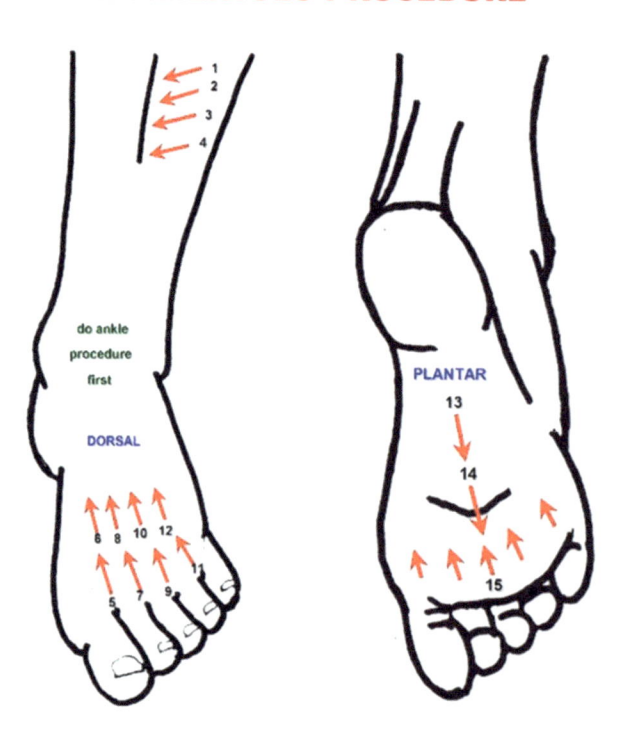

ANTERIOR TIBIAL PROCEDURE or Shin Procedure

Works for groin strains as well as foot pains

Prerequisites: Basic Relaxation Procedure 1, Hamstrings, Knee, Posterior Tibial

Procedure: Client in Supine position.

1. Left side 1st. Make 5 medial moves beginning inferior to the lateral tibial plateau down to the upper 1/3 of the tibia over the Anterior Tibial muscle.

ANTERIOR TIBIAL SHIN PROCEDURE

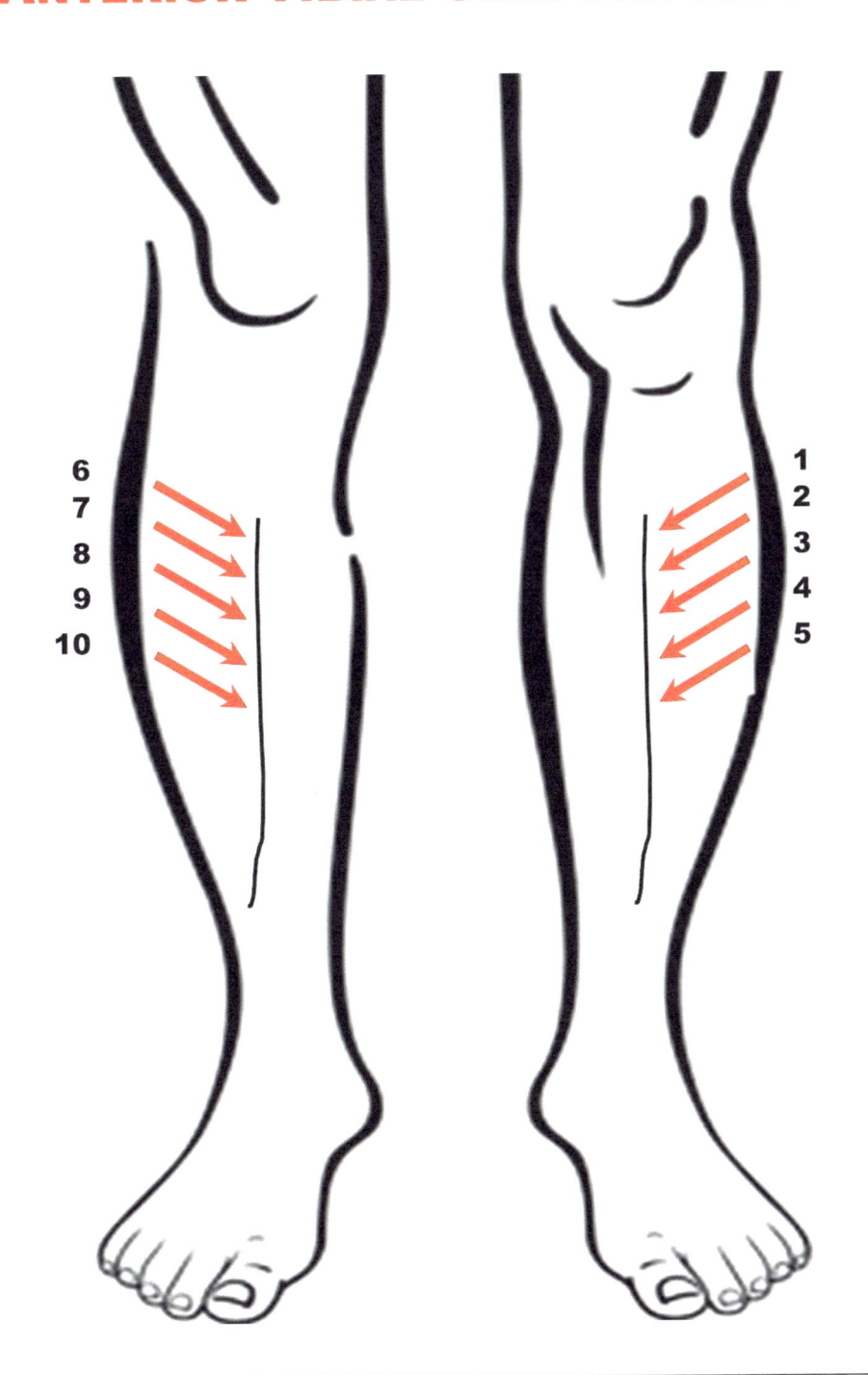

LONG EXTENSORS PROCEDURE

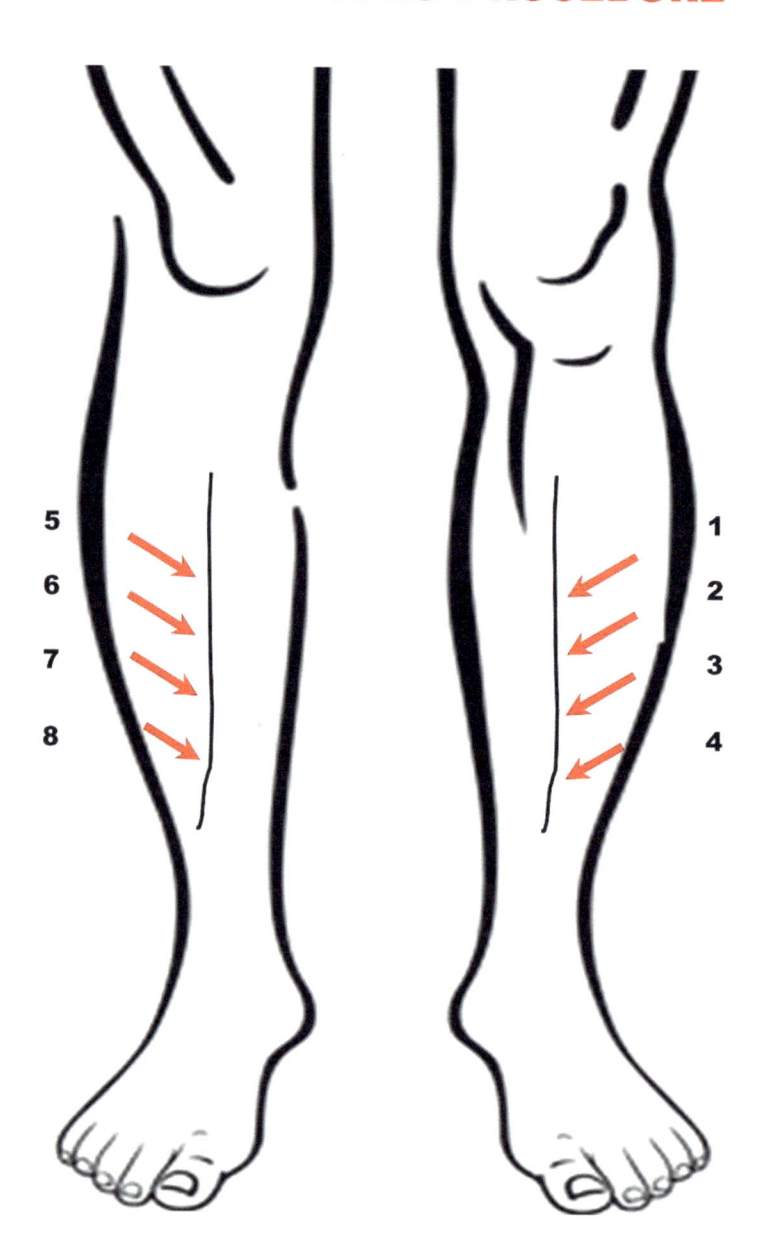

Prerequisites: Basic relaxation procedure 1, Hamstrings, Knee, Pelvis-anterior & posterior, Works best to follow with the Ankle Procedure.

Procedure: Client in prone position.

1. Moves 1 – 4: Medial moves over the EDL muscle. The proximal move is over the fibers to the 2nd toe. The distal move is over the fibers to the 5th toe. You can palpate the tendons on the dorsum of the foot corresponding to the muscle fibers being moved.

PERONEALS

Prerequisites: Basic Relaxation Procedure 1, Pelvis, Hamstrings, Knee

Procedure: Client in the supine position.

If there has been a history of ankle sprain/s or a present complaint of ITB problems, this is an important release point. Also check shoe wear for lateral heel skiving. Use when a client complains of numbness in the feet, or pain on the lateral foot area. Also suggested if there are problems with the hallux.

1. Make the moves 1 & 2 over the peroneus longus.
2. Move 3 over the peroneus brevis.
3. Move 4 over the peroneus tertius.

Peroneals Procedure

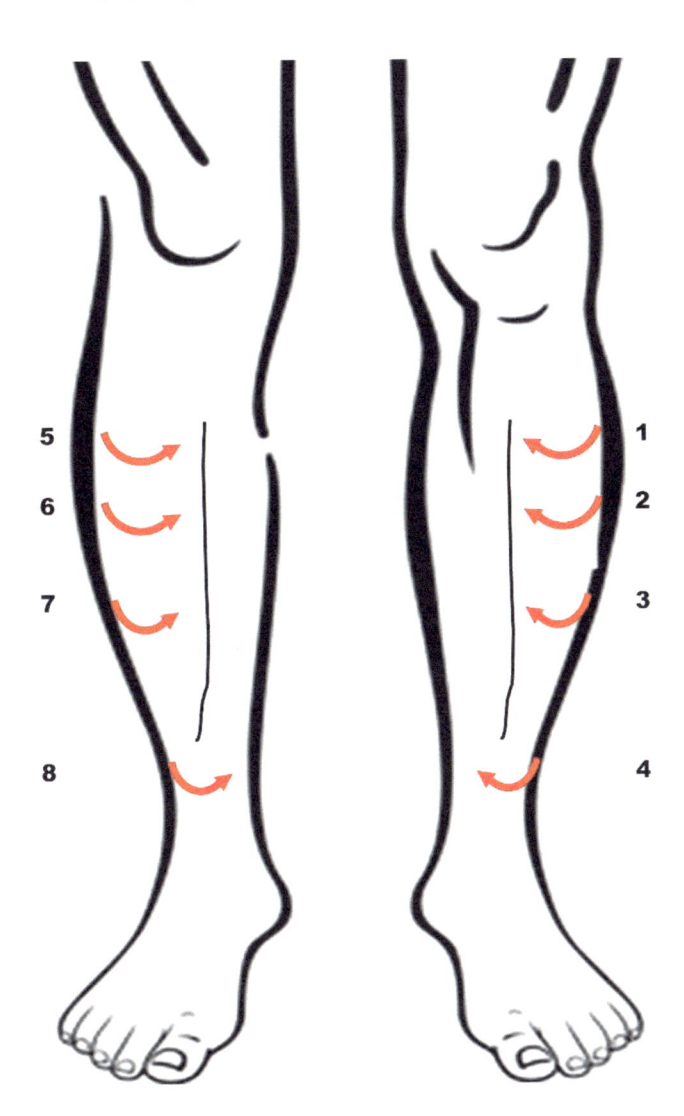

BUNION PROCEDURE

Prerequisites: Basic Relaxation Procedure 1 - Lower Back, Sacral, Coccyx, Sciatic 1 & 2, Anterior & Posterior pelvis, Long flexors, Long extensors, Ankle, Anterior tibial, Posterior tibial

Procedure: Client in prone position

1. Make a medial moves [1-2-3] with your thumb over the extensor hallusic longus tendon from the base of the 1st toe to the base of the 1st metatarsal.

2. Make 2 proximal moves [4] in the first intermetatarsal space.

3. Make a medial move [5] over the extensor hallusis longus tendon over the proximal phalanx.

4. Make 2 to 3 proximal to distal moves [6] across the adductor brevis muscle.

5. Make a plantar to dorsal move [7] over the abductor hallucis muscle.

6. Move the hallux in a circular direction and place a little traction on the joint.

BUNIONS PROCEDURE

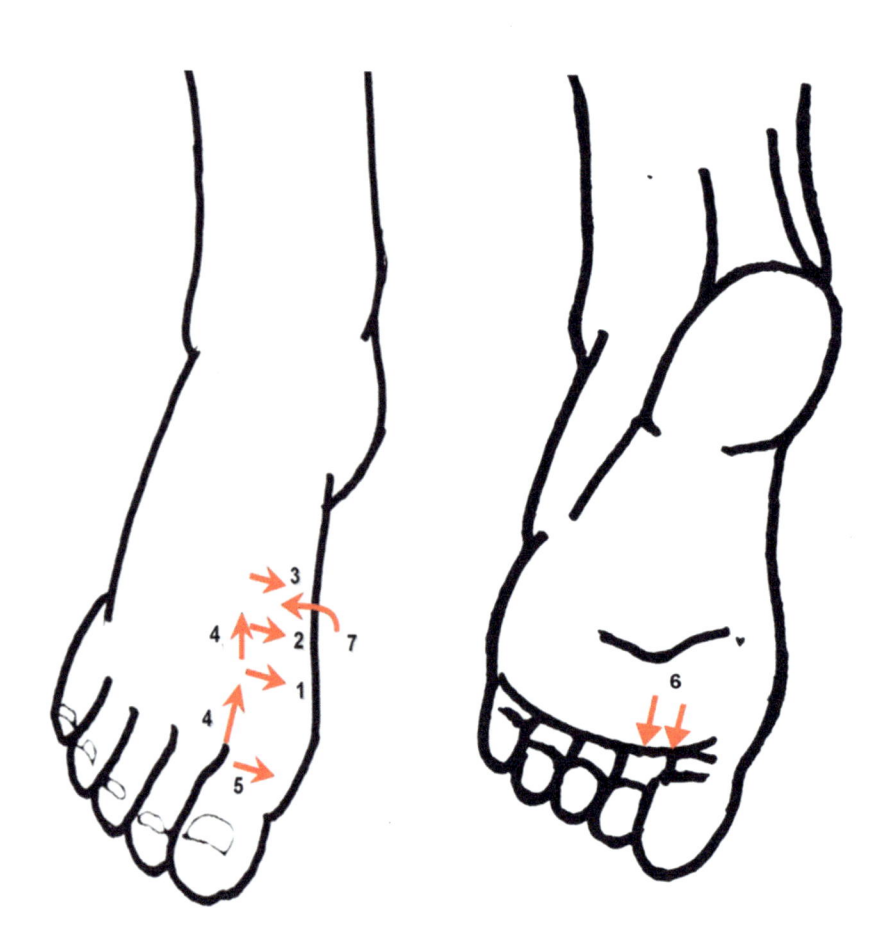

HEADACHE PROCEDURE

Prerequisites: None

Procedure: Client in a supine position. Practitioner at the head of the table

1. Place middle fingerpads at points 1 and hold for a count of 5 using mild pressure.
2. Continue to apply pressure while placing your index fingers on point 2 then release your middle fingers. Apply mild pressure to point 2 for 5 seconds.
3. Place thumbs on point 3 and apply mild pressure for 5 seconds while releasing fingers from point 2.
4. Place your ring fingers on point 4 and apply mild pressure for 5 seconds while releasing pressure on point 3.
5. Repeat 4 times.
6. Lastly, apply mild pressure over point 4 with the heels of hands for 10 seconds.
7. Allow client to rest for 10 to 15 minutes

HEADACHE PROCEDURE

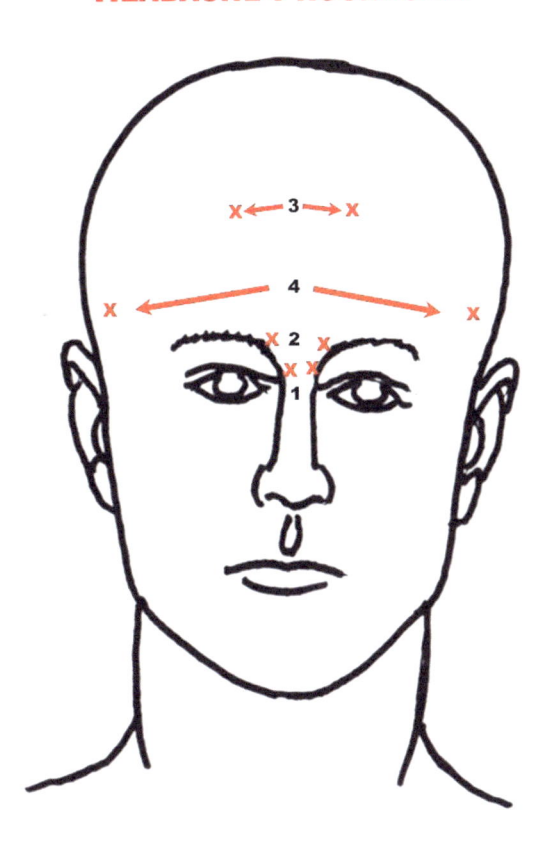

NECK PROCEDURE

Prerequisites: Basic Relaxation Procedures 1 and 2.

Procedure: Client in prone position.

Part A.

1. Perform moves 1 through 4 as in Neck Procedure 1. Wait 2 minutes minimum.

Part B.

2. Perform moves 5 and 6 as in Neck Procedure 1.
3. Make two additional medial moves above 5 & 6 = 7 and 8, and below moves 5 & 6 = 9 and 10.
4. Make 2 additional medial moves 11 and 12 over the Levator Scapula.
5. Moves 5 & 6 over the upper trapezius releases the neck.
6. Moves 7 & 8 above releases the TMJ area.
7. Moves 9 & 10 below releases the shoulder / arm areas.
8. Moves 11 & 12 release the shoulder area.

Neck Procedure

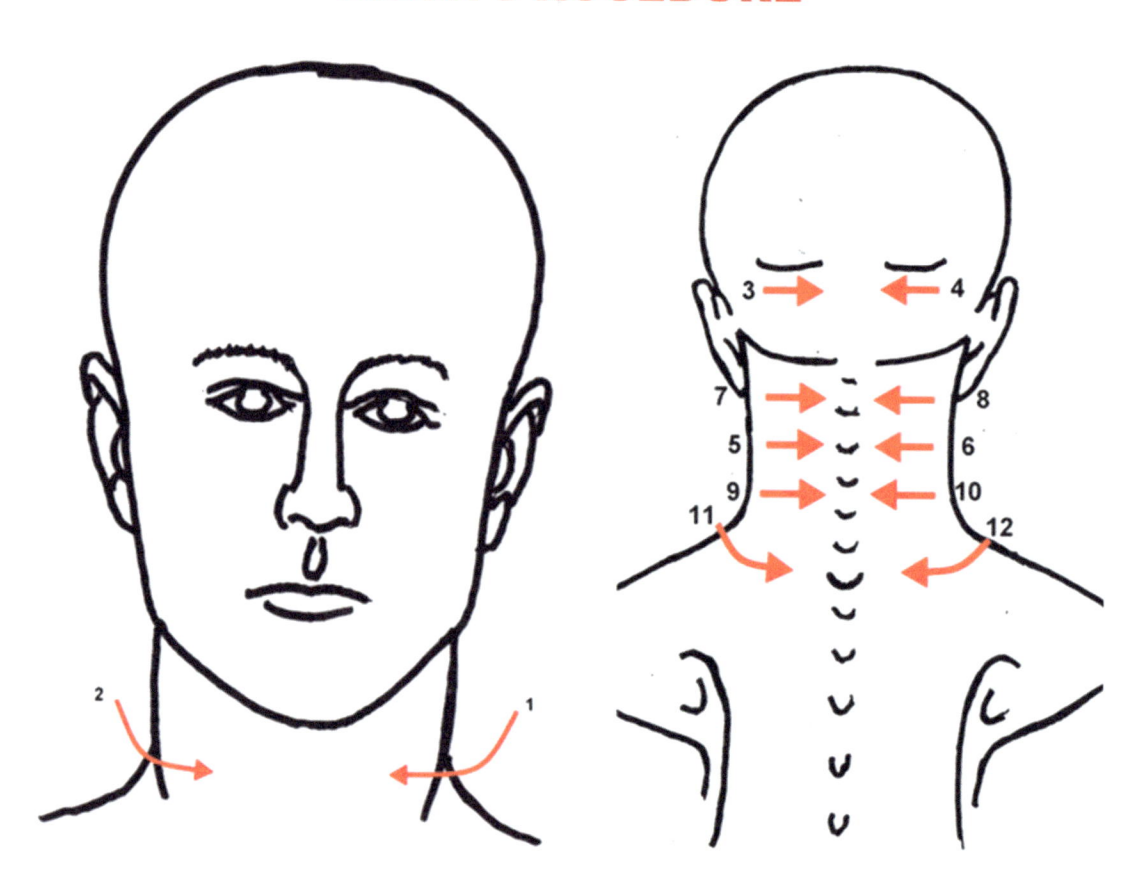

POSTERIOR PELVIS PROCEDURE

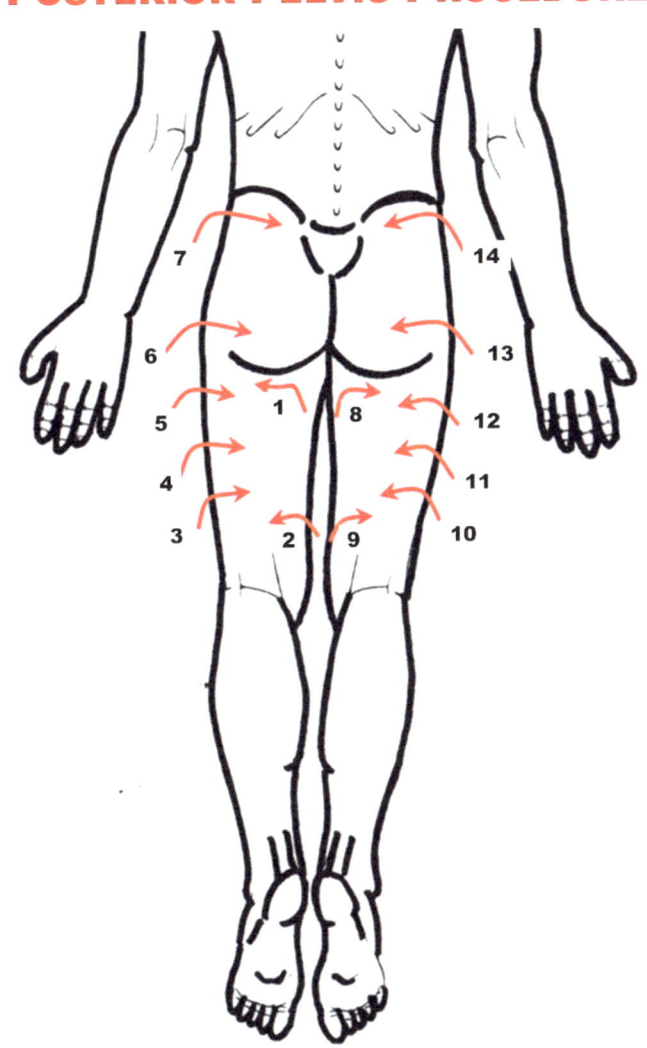

Prerequisites: Basic Relaxation Procedure 1

Procedure: Client in prone position. Left side first.

1. Move 1: Use your fingertips of your right hand. Push slack toward tabletop then make a posterior move over the Adductor Magnus.

2. Move 2: Use your middle finger right hand to push slack anterior then make a posterior move over the Adductor Magnus.

3. Moves 3 – 6: Use thumbs of both hands, push slack anteriorly and make moves posterior over the ITB.

4. Move 7: Use thumbs of both hands, push slack anteriorly and make a posterior move over the Tensor Fascia Lata.

POSTERIOR TIBIAL PROCEDURE

Prerequisites: Basic Relaxation Procedure 1, Hamstrings, Knee, Anterior Tibial

Procedure: Client in prone position. Left side 1st.

1. Bend the knee to 45 degrees flexion. Stabilize the lower leg.

2. Moves 1 – 3: Using your thumbs split the calf-lateral – medial. Wait 2 minutes.

3. Repeat moves 1 -3 if calf does not relax. Repeat until fully relaxed.

4. Move 4: Make a clockwise circle over the myotendinous junction of the Gastrocnemius & Soleus.

5. Moves 5 – 7: Make firm-deep lateral moves up the middle of the calf over the Posterior Tibial muscle. It is cord-like and may be tender. May repeat twice if needed.

POSTERIOR TIBIAL SHIN PROCEDURE

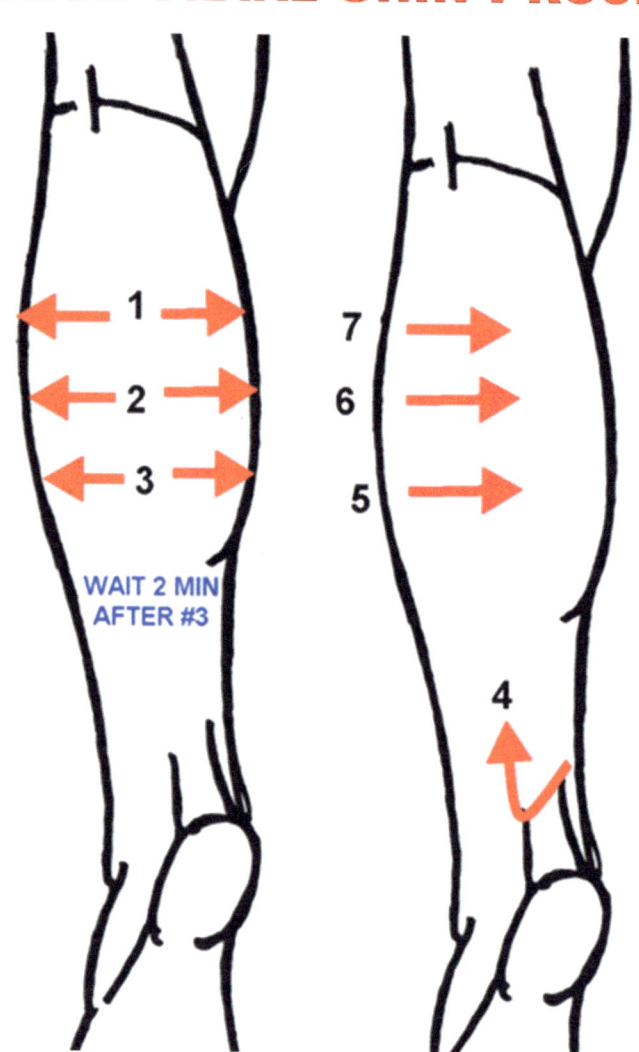

SACRAL / PREGNANT PROCEDURE

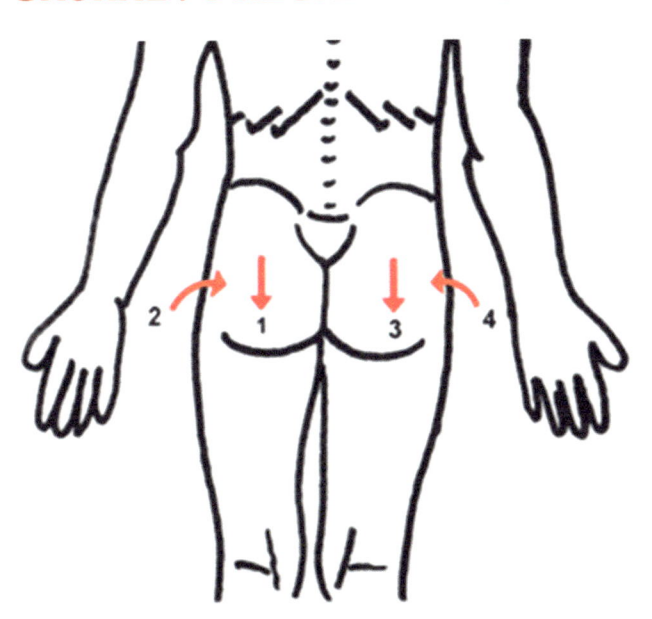

Prerequisites: Basic relaxation procedure 1. Moves 1 through 8

Procedure: Client in prone position. If pregnant, use big pillow, or perform standing [directions below].

Prone:

1. Practitioner on client's left side. Place right index finger over the reflex point in the coccyx procedure [approximately the top of the sacrum] on the left side, 1 inch from the midline. Remove slack superiorly and make an inferior move downward over the soft tissue spot with firm pressure to complete move 1.

2. Release your finger pressure for 5 seconds.

3. Replace your finger rotate your hand so the finger is pointing toward the spine on the reflex spot and hold with firm pressure.

4. With the thumb of your right hand remove slack over the tensor fascia latae posteriorly and make a firm anterior move over the tensor fascial latae, as was performed in moves 2 and 4 basic relaxation procedure 1, to complete move 2.

5. Repeat on right side with your left hand to complete moves 3 and 4.

Standing:

1. If pregnant lady, or other cannot lie on their stomach moves may be made while standing. Have client lean forward and support hands on countertop or an assistant while arching the neck forward and feet spread shoulder width. Make the moves as outlined above.

SACRAL / PREGNANT PROCEDURE

SCIATIC 1 PROCEDURE

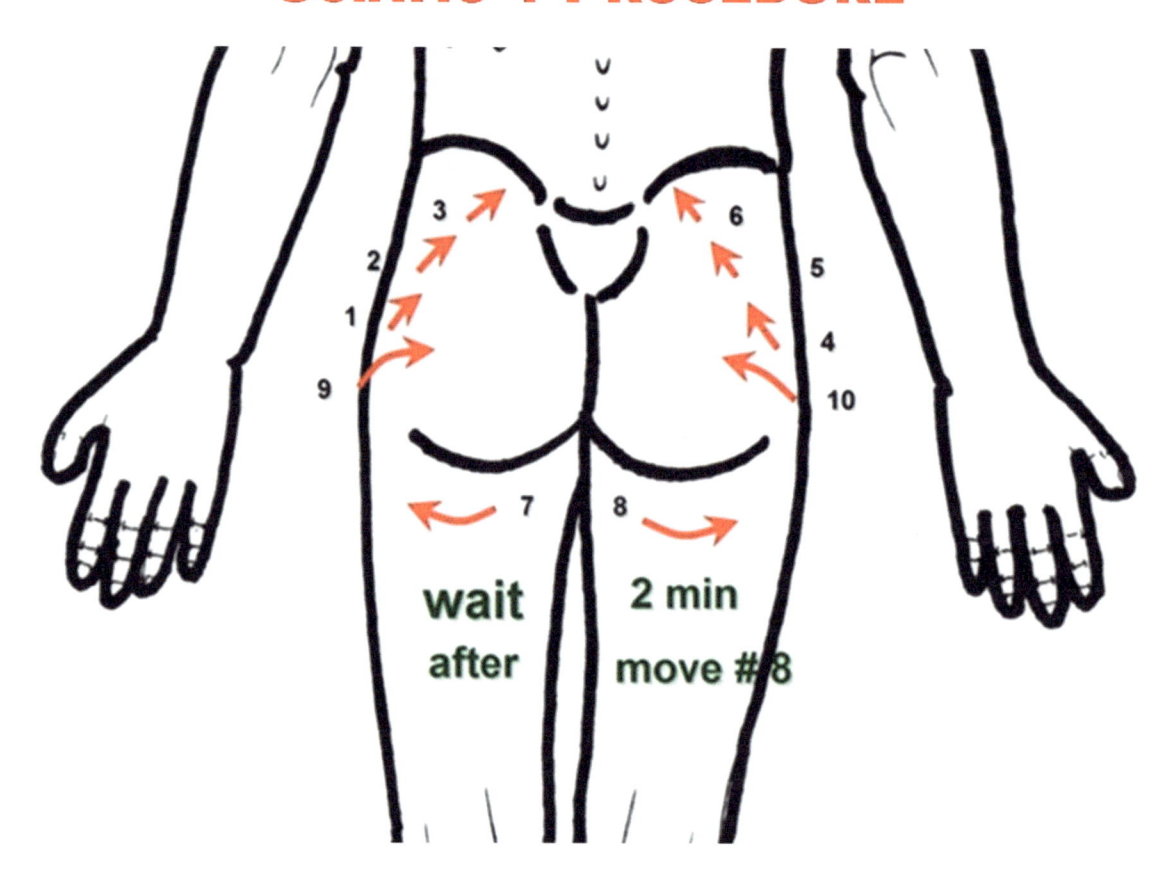

Prerequisite: None

Procedure: Left side first

2. Perform moves 1 through 8. Wait a minimum of 2 minutes.

3. Lift left leg 6 inches upward and abduct outward 6 inches.

4. Take slack laterally and make a firm move medial over the piriformis muscle. I use my thumb. You may use your elbow but be careful with the pressure.

5. Slowly return the leg to a resting position.

SCIATIC 2 PROCEDURE

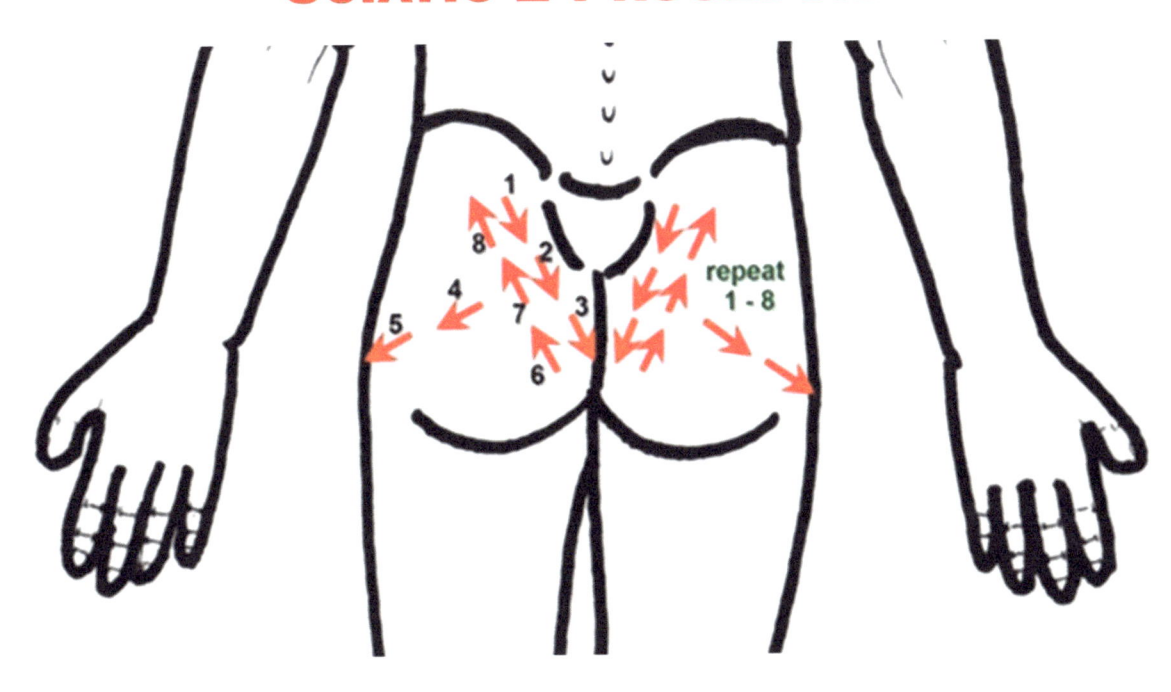

This procedure was developed by Albert LaShell, the late Milton Albrecht's cousin.

Prerequisite: Follow immediately after Hamstrings part A and before Kidney part B.

Procedure: Client is in the prone position.

1. Left side first. Abduct the leg about 6 inches.
2. Flex the knee to 90 degrees.
3. Holding the foot, adduct the foot which will internally rotate the hip. Holding at the end of the range of motion make moves 1 through 8.
4. Return leg to resting state and repeat on the right side.

SUBSTANCE DYSFUNCTION

N.A.E.T. [NAMBUDRIPAD's ALLERGY ELIMINATION TECHNIQUE]

AKA MOSHER'S - C.A.W.R. [CRAVINGS, ALLERGIES, WEIGHT, RESET]

A friend of mine who practices Naturopathy [natural healing with supplements, herbs, homeopathics, aroma therapy, essential oils, and other natural methods] told me of a technique she uses to remove allergic responses by the mind – body. She learned the technique from Dr. Devi Nambudripad, who is a chiropractor & acupuncturist. Devi accidentally discovered that by holding an allergen in the left hand and stimulating some acupoints along the bladder and governing vessel meridians, up the back and along the spine, the mind-body association can be broken. Another practitioner, who was a Bowen classmate, told me of a similar technique. If you know what you are allergic to, hold that in your left hand and shine a red laser light on an allergy point at the apex of the right ear for 30 seconds. Continue holding the substance for 20 minutes then discard it and do not come in contact with it for 25 hours. I asked. "Why 25 hours"? My friend told me that there are 12 main meridians which have 2 hour cycles during the 24 hour day. You do not know which meridian is affected by the allergen, and if you come in contact with the substance while the affected meridian is processing it will make you sick in some way or another.

My first experience was with the latter technique. Monday mornings I always sneezed and had a runny nose upon arriving at my office. I guessed that I was allergic to the toenail dust that is ever present in a podiatry office, even though we have vacuums attached to our nail drills. So, one Friday afternoon I caught some nail dust on a piece of adhesive tape. After patients I did the treatment and drove home holding the tape which took exactly 20 minutes. When I went to the office Monday and Tuesday I was unaware of anything different, then on Wednesday it occurred to me that I had done the allergy treatment the previous Friday and, that I had no runny nose or sneezing so far that week. As I write this, I no longer have any toenail dust symptoms. My second experience was with my friend Jean, our local naturopath who turned me on to this.

She determined that I was allergic to eggs, and when she told me so I recalled that whenever I ate eggs [which I really enjoyed] I felt very sluggish and spaced out the rest of the day. After she did the N.A.E.T. clearing on me I have had no further symptoms after eating eggs. My third significant experience came from a self-treatment which turned out to be rather bazaar. I learned that I was allergic to sillymarin and rosemary, both of which were in my multiple vitamins. One afternoon I used the laser light on the ear point technique, held on to the vitamin tablet for 20 minutes, then discarded it. The following morning I made sure not to take the multiple vitamins which had not passed the 25 hour mark, so I took all of my other morning supplements. I was in a bit of a hurry so I didn't fix anything for breakfast but got a piece of leftover fish from the fridge and was on my way. When I arrived at my office, all of a sudden I felt like I'd been hit by a truck. I got achy, my head pounded, and my nose bled. We had to cancel my morning appointments and I laid down for a rest. When I awakened at 11:00 AM I felt better, and as I got up I detected a strange taste in my mouth. *ROSEMARY!* The fish had been breaded with seasoned bread crumbs and I ingested them as the stomach meridian was cycling [7:00 – 9:00 AM].

Another twisted, bazaar, and unusual case occurred with a patient of mine. She was diagnosed with Morton's neuroma [enlarged nerve] between the 3rd and 4th metatarsals. This is a fairly common foot condition, and I feel quite proficient in its diagnosis and treatment. She had the usual numbness, tingling, and occasional burning in her 2nd, 3rd, & 4th toes in both feet. I performed my usual and customary non-surgical treatments and she seemed to improve. I the made her orthotics to keep pressure from the nerves and instructed her to return in 2 months if any problems still occurred and I would discuss surgical treatment. 2 years hence a friend of hers was seeing me for a problem, and she told me the rest of the story. Apparently my patient with the neuromas experienced progression of symptoms up the ankles and legs. Her family doctor referred her to a neurologist who diagnosed Multiple Sclerosis and prescribed drugs for this. She went to Stanford for a 2nd opinion and was again diagnosed with M.S. She tried other medications which did not help. Then, a year or so later it began affecting her hands. At this point she went to the Mayo Clinic, and again she was diagnosed with M.S., and was given some other medications. About the time she lost the use of her thumbs, she went to my naturopath friend, Jean. After Jean completed her work-up she was surprised that the lady did not show any of the usual findings that go along with neuropathies. She then asked our patient about what was happening in her life when all of this began. As it turns out she was building her dream home at the time of a real estate slump, and she was the not so proud owner of 2 spec. houses which were not selling. All kinds of stress were abundant in her life at the time. She recalled the first sign of the tingling in her toes when she walked bare footed across the Mexican paver's tile in the hallway. Jean then tested her for allergy to the tile, and sure enough, she was. Within days following a clearing her symptoms began to reverse, and within a month she was totally symptom free. However, as soon as she went back to walking on the tile floor the tingling in the toes returned so, she ended up selling the house.

I surmise that the process works like this. Let's assume that you have never been in contact with rosemary. During a time of stress and duress you eat your first dose of rosemary. From then on your mind, [cell membranes], associates rosemary with stress. And, whenever you come in contact with rosemary the mind, [cell membranes] tells the body and the body goes into a stress pattern. Depending on which meridian was initially affected symptoms will be the same, each time of exposure. This is a different type of allergy than the poison oak type, whereby the substance causes the formation of antibodies which attack the allergen and thus cause an inflammatory reaction. So, I call this phenomenon, SUBSTANCE DYSFUNCTION.

I have incorporated this concept into the Bowen Therapy session on a number of occasions, myself included. Believe it or not, I eliminated cravings for potatoe chips and crackers with cheese a couple of months ago. My theory is that we crave what we are allergic or sensitive to. Therefore, I held these items written on a piece of paper [after all, if the ice crystal experiments by Emoto responded to the vibratory rate of the written word, so should this], while having a session. I have only eaten not craved, chips on 2 to 3 occasions and zero crackers and cheese for over 2 months. I used to need these on a daily basis. Now that my body has experienced this change I am going to tackle another craving in a few weeks.

For patients, I have performed this for all kinds of actual food allergies as well as emotional holdings, and it almost always works. How it really works is beside me, but I remember that my patients really only care if it works, not how. For those of us who must have an explanation- I propose one - which surfaced since I wrote the above for this manuscript I am in the process of writing. I stumbled on to a book titled, "The Molecules of Emotion", by Candace Pert, Ph.D. She points out that endorphins [our very own narcotic/tranquilizer substance], is in part, contained in the nodal points along the spine, [see chapter 4 for complete list].These are the precise locations for many of the Bowen moves. My patients tell me quite often that during the day following their treatment they felt a kind of "Runner's High", and for the remainder of the week a sense of well-being. Dr. Pert further discovered that the endorphins are one of the mechanisms by which the immune, central, and endocrine systems network with each other. In other words, the mind-body connection, maybe. So, if you have a negative mind- body connection to a food, chemical, substance, or color that becomes a stressor and the meridian system will react to the stimulus of it. If you hold that same substance in your left hand in the presence of endorphin release that substance is now equated with a sense of well being and the old negative program is cancelled out. In some circles it is accepted that one craves what one is allergic to, i.e. alcohol.

If you have followed my logic so far, hang in there for the next two scenarios, because these are huge, [no pun intended]. Weight control and sugar!!

THE SUGAR CONNECTION

After breast milk, one of the first substances we come into contact with is *SUGAR!* If there is a moderate amount of stress and turmoil during infancy, there is a strong likelihood that sugar may turn out to be a stressing substance for that individual throughout the years. I have released the craving for sugar in a number of my adult patients. I am looking forward to doing a study on children for the release of the sugar connection.

THE WEIGHT CONNECTION

Have you ever pondered why there is such a yo-yo effect with dieting? I have. My conclusions are; that there are emotional fulfillments by the ingestion of certain foods in different individuals, and our subconscious has a body mass – weight, "set point", which it tries very hard to maintain. Therefore, your conscious mind says, "I need to lose 30 pounds for my upcoming class reunion". So you do, but 3 months after the reunion, the weight is all back, maybe plus some. Your subconscious guides you to eat those foods and quantities of foods which will take you back to the weight where it is "set". Wouldn't it be nice to develop a new "set points" so that you can eat your way to weight-loss? The conscious – sub-conscious awareness is an enigma. How many times have you disregarded your gut feeling, intuition, and instant recall processes, and found out later on that your conscious and logical thinking talked you out of the right answer? My theory is, "If you can eliminate those foods and substances which you crave [including sugar], and once a month re-program a new set *point*, 5 pounds or less lighter, than the existing one", you will lose weight, maintain. Weight Watchers, South Beach, Eat 4 Your Blood Type, etc. programs, and may be better able to keep the weight off over the long haul.

I HAVE RESET THE FOLLOWING IN SOME OF MY PATIENTS:

- Sugar
- Chips
- Crackers
- Sodas
- Marijuana
- Red wine
- Shellfish
- Chocolates
- Weight
- Cookies and cakes
- Anger

Finally, Dr. Bruce Lipton, in his book titled, THE BIOLOGY OF BELIEF, refers to studies he performed in laboratory experiments which discovered that the cell's membrane is not only a filter and protective barrier, but a silicon chip. The membrane [Brane =Brain], takes in data, processes the data, stores the data, and releases important information to adjacent cells, tissues, and systems. The cell's membrane contains hundreds of receptor sites for neurotransmitters and hormones which all compete for keys which fit those locks. Some keys look like other keys and the receptor sites will take up those keys. For example, D.D.T. & D.E.S. are very close to Estrogen in their molecular configuration. So, the receptor does not know the exact difference between the 3, and might allow one of the D.D.T. or D.E.S. in!! Same as, the receptor site for endorphin cannot differentiate between endorphin and morphine. Both are similar in molecular configuration, so they compete for a site of attachment- Morphine usually wins!!

So, if I could send a new signal to the cell's membranes that substance "A" was okay-the cell's membrane recognized this - and stored it. Would it not be within the realm of possibility that substance "A", was now recognized as a friendly, rather than an adversary. Now, when substance "A" comes into the scene, the cells do not over-react.

How to determine what your client is allergic to:

1. Enterro / E.A.V. [Electro Acupuncture by Voll.
2. QXCI.
3. Applied Kinesiology / Muscle Testing.
4. By history of the client.

How to perform the ReSet:

1. Have client hold the substance or the written description of it in their left hand. This can be done to clear known emotional holdings as well.

2. Perform a full Basic Bowen sequence; BRP 1 – BRP 2 – KIDNEY – LOWER RESPIRATORY [AKA ASTHMA] – HAMSTRINGS – BRP 3 – KIDNEY – ANTERIOR PELVIS – ANKLE – UPPER RESPITATORY [AKA HAY FEVER ALLERGY] – TMJ, as they hold the substance, or paper with writing. The session should last about 1 hour - so plenty of long rests for the body to process.

3. Advise patient to avoid the stimulus that they are clearing for 25 hours just to be safe. Prepare them for any adverse psychosomatic reactions which may rarely occur, [emotional release, increased pain, new pain, old pain].

The following are the experiences of Dr. Mitchell Mosher utilizing Bowen Therapy for specific ailments or injuries. These are his clinical observations.

ALLERGY / SENSITIVITY CLEARING

The next experience was with toenail dust. In the grinding down process of thinning patients thick nails a good deal of dust is created. For safety we used vacuums attached to the drills, but there was always a little residue. I collected some dust on a piece of tape and took it to my Bowen associate. I had her do the Bowen moves up my spine over the erector muscles while holding the tape in my left hand. From then on, I didn't experience the usual sneezing and runny nose when I got to the office on Monday mornings like I used to.

After moving to North Carolina I started getting seasonal hay fever and allergies. These were most pronounced in the fall and winter. A few weeks ago while working outdoors near Lake Wylie the allergies began again. There was a stiff breeze blowing off the lake and I had a flash-back of the tape and toe nail dust incident many years ago. I pinned a piece of duct tape on the wall of the shop adhesive side facing the breeze and the lake. The next morning the piece of tape was taken to my Bowen therapist and she did the moves as instructed.

When I got off of the table there was a complete clearing of all the symptoms. My nose wasn't running as it was before and remain symptom free three weeks later.

OTHER CONSIDERATIONS:

A Naturopathic practitioner named Gene, who was a Bowen classmate, told me of a technique to remove allergies. He told me that if you know what you are allergic to, you can hold that substance in your left hand and shine a red laser light on the allergy point at the apex of the right ear for 30 seconds. Then, continue holding the substance for 20 minutes, and then discard it, but don't come in contact with it for 25 hours. I asked. "Why 25 hours?" My friend told me that there are 12 main meridians which have 2 hour cycles during the 24 hour day. You don't know which meridian is affected by the allergen, and if you come in contact with the substance while the affected meridian is processing it will make you sick in some way or another. You'll see when you come to the Rosemary part.

My first experience with the technique proceeded as follows. Monday mornings I always sneezed and got a runny nose upon arriving at my office. I guessed that I was allergic to the toenail dust that is ever present in a podiatry office, even though we have vacuums attached to our nail drills. So, one Friday afternoon I caught some nail dust on a piece of adhesive tape. After patients I did the treatment with the helium beam on my CO2 laser and drove home holding the tape, which took exactly 20 minutes. When I went to the office Monday and Tuesday, I was unaware of anything different. Then on Wednesday, it occurred to me that I had done the allergy treatment the previous Friday and, that I had no runny nose or sneezing so far that week. As I write this, I no longer have any toenail dust symptoms.

N.A.E.T. Nambudripad's Allergy Elimination Technique

A friend of mine who practices Naturopathy - natural healing with supplements, herbs, homeopathy, aroma therapy, essential oils, and other natural methods, told me of a technique she uses to remove allergic responses by the mind – body. Dr. Devi Nambudripad is an RN., Chiropractor & Acupuncturist. Dr. Devi accidentally discovered that by holding an allergen in the left hand and stimulating some acupoints along the bladder and governing vessel meridians, up the back and along the spine, the mind-body association can be repaired or replaced. Her book is titled, "SAY GOODBYE TO ILLNESS". N.A.E.T. is an acronym for, "Nambudripad's Allergy Elimination Technique".

My Naturopathic friend Jean, determined that I was allergic to eggs, plus some other things. When she told me so, I recalled that whenever I ate eggs, which I really enjoyed, I felt very sluggish and spaced out the rest of the day until around 4:00 PM. After she did the N.A.E.T. clearing on me, I've had no further symptoms after eating eggs.

Case Study: Rosemary – A lesson in the body processing process.

My third significant experience came from a self-treatment which turned out to be rather bizarre. I learned that I was allergic to silymarin and rosemary, both of which were in my multiple vitamins. One afternoon I used the laser light on the ear point technique, held on to the vitamin tablet for 20 minutes, then discarded it. The following morning, I made sure not to take the multiple vitamins which had not passed the 25-hour mark, so I took all of my other morning supplements. I was in a bit of a hurry so I didn't fix anything for breakfast but grabbed a piece of leftover fish from the fridge, and was on my way. When I arrived at my office, all of a sudden, I felt like I'd been hit by a truck. I got achy, my head pounded, I got chilled, and my nose bled. We had to cancel my morning appointments. I laid down for a rest on one of my massage tables and covered with a blanket. When I awoke at 11:00 AM, I felt better. And, as I got up, I detected a strange taste in my mouth. *ROSEMARY!* The fish had been breaded with *seasoned* bread crumbs and I ingested them as the stomach meridian was cycling from 7:00 – 9:00 AM.

An unusually interesting case occurred with a patient of mine. It has nothing to do with Bowen Therapy, but I am including it so that someone's may benefit from the information. I diagnosed her foot problem with Morton's neuroma, which is an enlarged nerve between the 3rd and 4th metatarsals. This is a fairly common foot condition, and I felt quite proficient in its diagnosis and treatment options. She had the usual numbness, tingling, and occasional burning in her 2nd, 3rd, & 4th toes in both feet. I performed my usual and customary non-surgical treatments and she seemed to improve. I the made her orthotics to keep pressure from the nerves and instructed her to return in two months if any problems still occurred and we would discuss surgical treatment.

About two years hence a friend of hers was seeing me for a problem, and she told me the rest of the story. Apparently, my patient with the neuromas experienced progression of symptoms up the ankles and legs. Her family doctor referred her to a neurologist who diagnosed Multiple Sclerosis and prescribed drugs for this. She went to Stanford University for a 2nd opinion, and was again diagnosed with M.S. She tried other medications which did not help. Then, a year or so later it began affecting her hands. At this point she went to the Mayo Clinic in Arizona, and again she was diagnosed with M.S., and was given some other medications. About the time she lost the use of her thumbs, she went to my naturopath friend, Jean.

After Jean completed her work-up she was surprised that the lady did not show any of the usual findings that go along with neuropathies. She then asked our patient about what was happening in her life when all of this began. As it turns out she was building her dream home at the time of a real estate slump, and she was the not so proud owner of two houses built on speculation, which were not selling. All kinds of stress were abundant in her life at the time. She recalled the first sign of the tingling in her toes when she walked bare footed across the Mexican paver's tile in the hallway of the new home. Jean then tested her for allergy to the tile, and sure enough, she was. Within days following a clearing her symptoms began to reverse, and within a month she was totally symptom free. However, as soon as she went back to walking on the tile floor the tingling in the toes returned so, she ended up selling the house

N.A.E.T. MY INTERPRETATION

I got thinking one day about the N.A.E.T. technique. It occurred to me that many of the Bowen Therapy moves are over the same meridian points along the spine.

I discussed my allergy theory with a patient whom I was doing some Bowen sessions on. Her 12-year-old son had multiple allergies and was seeing the local allergist for allergy shots. One of his main allergens was shellfish. If he ate any shellfish whatsoever, he suffered laryngospasms and hives. He also often craved shellfish. The allergist was afraid to give him allergy shots for shellfish for fear of a serious reaction. I had mother bring him for a Bowen session during which I had him hold a shrimp in his left hand during the treatment. When mother came back the following week she told me that his allergy skin test for shellfish had reduced by 80%. Unfortunately, they moved to Texas shortly after, so I did not get to follow up with them.

Emotional clearing with Bowen / N.A.E.T.

Although this experience did not involve a substance, I include It because it seems to be relevant. My naturopath friend Jean, referred me a patient that she was having trouble keeping cleared of the issues which were causing her headaches. Jean suspected that there might be an emotional block that was keeping her from attaining lasting relief. The patient had an anger issue with her father. It came from an incident when she was five years old. Her father and his friend went duck hunting and locked her in the car at the hunting spot for about four hours. She recalls the fright and feeling of abandonment which resulted in a long and deep anger toward her father. Although she had forgiven him and was at peace on a conscious level, she knew that there was some inner resentment that lingered. The first Bowen session, my intent was for me to initiate a somatic-emotional release if that was what she needed. Nothing happened. The next visit, on a hunch, I had her write her desire to be rid of the anger toward father on a piece of paper. She held it in her left hand while I performed a full Bowen session on her. She returned a week later and was over it. She had experienced two days of extreme anger, especially with her two children. She was a single mom who doted over her kids, and hardly ever got upset with them. But, for the two days just about everything they did or said upset her. The last I heard, she was still pain free, and her life was good.

Other Cases of interest.

Another of my patients mentioned that whenever she drank a glass of red wine, she developed a panic attack right after. This didn't happen to her with white wine. However, she didn't like white wine. She only liked red. So, we wrote red wine on a post-it note. She held this in her left hand while I did an abbreviated Bowen session using procedures 1-2-3. When she returned a month later for her Bowen "Tune-up", she was no longer sensitive to red wine.

A friend of mine began experiencing headaches after drinking only a sip of red wine. I performed the same clearing for him, and he has been fine ever since.

My naturopath friend, Jean had a client who she was treating. She suffered headaches during the week. But, not on the weekends. After it was all said and done, Jean found that her client was sensitive to the color orange. She worked for Cal Trans and they had to wear orange vests while at work on the freeways and roads in California. She had the option to wear purple instead, and as soon as she switched colors, her chronic headaches cleared.

Another interesting case occurred recently at the cancer clinic where I used to do therapy. Mandy had sugar cravings, and I cleared her of those. Then she told me that she was unable to tolerate fried eggs. She could eat eggs in any other form, but she vomited after eating fried eggs. I did the clearing, and she now can eat fried eggs with no problem.

Cravings.

I was moderately addicted to potato chips. I always ate a small bag on my way home from work. I went to the pantry soon after arriving home and got more chips, and then some more. This went on most every day. After a hypnotherapy session, I was okay with it for a couple of years, but the cravings came back. I wrote potato chips on a small piece of paper and had a Bowen session with a practitioner whom I traded with. The same day I drove home empty handed. When I got home I did not feel even slightly inclined to go to the pantry and get some chips! To this day, some 15 years hence, I don't crave potato chips at all.

One of my Bowen patients confessed to craving diet sodas. She drank upward to 12 a day. We wrote "diet soda pop" on a piece of paper and did her Bowen session as she held the paper in her left hand. When she returned the following week, she had not had but three diet sodas all week. The next week she had none!

Other cravings eliminated in patients: Marijuana, Sugar, Chocolates, Coffee

Has not been shown to work for nicotine.

THE SUGAR CONNECTION

After breast milk, one of the first substances we come into contact with is *SUGAR!* If there is a moderate amount of stress and turmoil during infancy, there is a possibility that sugar may turn out to be a stressing substance for that individual throughout the years. I have released the craving for sugar in a number of my adult patients. I am looking forward to doing a study on children for the release of the sugar connection. My theory is, that this disconnection process to sugar may be responsible to ADD and ADHD. I surmise that we all might be afflicted by the sugar connection to some degree. It may be possible, that the more the stress was at first contact, the greater the subsequence reactions

How can any of this be possible?

My theory is that the process works like this. First, let's assume that you have never been in contact with root beer. Then during a time of stress and duress you eat your first dose of root beer. From now on your mind associates root beer with stress. And, even though you now are stress free, whenever you come in contact with root beer the body goes into a stress reaction pattern. Depending on which meridian was initially affected symptoms will be the same each time of exposure to root beer. I may be sensitive to root beer and experience headaches from it. You may be sensitive to root beer and you experience diarrhea when you come in contact with it. This is a different type of allergy than the poison oak type, whereby the substance causes the formation of antibodies which attack the allergen and thus cause an inflammatory reaction.

Secondly, my problem with eggs came from my stint in the U.S. Army. I ate eggs for breakfast at least five days a week. I was under stress for most of the two years I served. I was home-sick, love-sick, overworked, underpaid, harassed by the "Officers." I remember eating eggs while in high school without any problems. But they affected me my entire adult life, until Jean did the clearing for me. So, it was a repeated exposure over a long-time frame under stress in this instance.

For patients, I have performed this for all kinds of actual food allergies as well as emotional holdings, and it almost always works. How it really works is beside me, but I remember that my patients really only care if it works, not how. For those of us who must have an explanation, I propose one. I stumbled on to a book titled, "The Molecules of Emotion:", by Candace Pert, Ph.D. She points out that endorphins which are our very own narcotic/tranquilizer substance, are in part, contained in the nodal points along the spine. These are the precise locations for many of the Bowen moves. My patients tell me quite often that during the Bowen session and the day following their treatment, they felt a kind of "Runner's High", and for the remainder of the week a sense of well-being. Dr. Pert further discovered that the endorphins are one of the mechanisms by which the immune, central, and endocrine systems network with each other. In other words, the mind-body connection, maybe. So, if you have a negative mind- body connection to a food, chemical, substance, or color that becomes a stressor and the meridian system will react to the stimulus of it. If you hold that same substance in your left hand in the presence of endorphin release that substance is now equated with a sense of wellbeing and the old negative program is cancelled out, or over-ridden. In some circles it is accepted that one craves what one is allergic to, i.e. sugar / alcohol.

Why would any changes take place from merely holding something written on a piece of paper? If the ice crystal experiments by Masuro Emoto responded to the vibratory rate of the written word in his experiments. Maybe that's why this has had some influence on patients while having a Bowen Medical Bodywork session?

ANKLE SPRAINS

I attended an advanced Bowen workshop one weekend and talked with a classmate about our experiences during the previous months performing the therapy. He told me that he'd treated a number of football players at the University of California, Berkeley with acute ankle sprains with the, " Ankle Procedure". He was doing this immediately after the injury. I was amazed that he could do this in spite of pain and swelling that follows an ankle sprain.

The following Monday morning, a father brought his 14-year-old daughter in who'd sprained her ankle playing soccer on Saturday. Her ankle was extremely swollen, ecchymosed (bruised), and painful. She was using crutches for ambulation and had an ace bandage wrapped around the ankle. Following my examination, which only confirmed the obvious, I thought to myself, "Here goes nothing", and I began a Bowen session. I explained to father that the muscles enter a state of spasm following the trauma to guard the tissues from further injury, and this can perpetuate pain and swelling. When it came time to do the "ankle procedure" following relaxation of all of the leg and thigh muscles, I noticed butterflies in my stomach. I moved the anterior tibial tendon medially. Then I slid my fingers over the lateral malleolus and posterior over the lateral collateral and my thumb over the deltoid ligament. As I dorsiflexed and plantar flexed the first metatarsal my thoughts turned to the last part of the procedure which strikes the ball of the foot to, "Set" the ankle." Much to my surprise, she didn't flinch as I struck the M-P joints with my closed fist.

I invited her to stand up on her feet. Following, which she walked out of the room quite normally and said, "Oh dad. You grab the crutches." I gulped, and thought, "Hooray, it worked!"

ARTHRITIS

One of my more interesting experiences occurred with a patient and his responses, which took place the very first week I started doing Bowen. Another Podiatrist down the road who was not able to help him referred Bernard to me. Bernard had an arthritic large toe joint, which he did not want to have surgery on. He told me that he was favoring the toe and this was making his hip and back painful. He was hopeful that some type of shoe modification would suffice to relieve his problems. His joint was red, swollen, tender, and with movement grated like sand paper crepitus. I informed him that I could accommodate his shoe and for him to leave it over the weekend and I would get it done. Then I also told him about the Bowen treatment, which might relieve the pains in his hip and back. He begged me to also perform the upper back and neck moves and promised he wouldn't tell anyone. this was before I obtained a massage certificate- rermember, my podiatry license only covered the leg muscles. I felt comfortable with him, so I did a complete treatment from head to toe. When I had finished the procedures that I had learned in class, I examined his Extensor Hallucis Longus muscles, the muscle that draws the big toe upward. The one on the right side was like a rope. So, I figured that if they had taught a procedure on this in class, it would be slack to the table and make an anterior move, good side first. So, I worked on the left side 1st, and then did the right side muscle, and he immediately let out a moan. I asked if he was all right, and he said, "I'm alright. It kind of hurt and tickled at the same time".

I left the room for a few minutes in order to let him rest and for the release to take place. When I returned, he was curled up in a fetal position and was quite pale and cold. My first thought was that he'd fainted and was going into shock. I checked his pulse and was going to take his blood pressure when he said," I'm okay. I'm a little cold. May I have a blanket?" I covered him up and left him alone to settle down for a few minutes. The rest of his story is in th emotional clearing section . I gave him his post-treatment instructions and told him to pick up his shoe on Monday.

When I saw him on seated in the waiting room Monday morning prior to appointment times I said, "Hi Bernard. I've got your shoe ready". He said very emphatically, "I don't care about the shoe. I want to know when I can get another treatment?" I said, "That's right, I gave you a Bowen last week. How'd it work?" He said, "How'd it work? It changed my life! The past 3 nights have been the only full night's sleep I have had in years. My back doesn't hurt. The pain in my hip is all but gone and look at my toe!". He commenced to remove his shoe and sock and bent the toe up and down and said, "See. Look at this". I couldn't help but walk out into the waiting room and look at his toe up close. The swelling, redness and crepitus were completely resolved. There remained a little stiffness, but the toe flexed at least 50% more than it did on Friday. I told him that he could make an appointment for Friday.

BACK PAIN: Lower

My low back pain had increasing and more frequently occurring. This had been going on for about 12 years. I had been to my family doctor, physical therapists, chiropractors, massage therapists, acupuncturists, and so on over the years and I thought that I had exhausted my conservative options, and that I was going to need the neurosurgeon. A patient told me about the late Milton Albrecht who performed this Bowen Technique so I decided to give Bowen a try. I was elated to find that my back pain and four different foot and leg problems resolved following a solitary treatment. The cause of my back pain was coming from a tight leg muscle! No wonder my back didn't get better when all the practitioners were working on my back. (More)

Out of 15,000 or so patients I have done Bowen sessions for since 1995, at least 20% had low back pain. I did a pain study shortly before I retired from my podiatry practice. Patients graded their pain on a scale of 1 to 10 - 10 = severe, 1 = mild. I was going to write a paper on the results, but retirement got in the way. So, I'm going to use my recall to tell you the results. Within three weekly sessions, 50% were resolved. Following three more monthly sessions, 80% were resolved or improved.

BACK PAIN: UPPER

Jenny came to my office with a sprained ankle. She'd been to one of those "Doc in a Box" places, and was placed in a removable cast boot. Because it was lifting her up about one inch on the left side, her back and hip was painful. She wanted to know if there were any other options. I splinted her ankle with adhesive tape and gave her a Bowen session. I later found out that she'd had a standing appointment at her chiropractor's office every Friday at 4:00 PM to treat her upper back and shoulder pain. She was in the janitorial business and apparently was straining these muscles repeatedly. However, following just two Bowen sessions she no longer had to go to the chiropractor. After four weeks absence, he called her to see if she was all right. When she told him had happened, he hung up on her.

She was came back to my office for another problem a few years later, and I asked her about her shoulder/back problem. She'd not had a pain in over nine years even though she still does the same kind of work.

BED WETTING

The few dozen times I've used the technique, it has resolved the issue. It does involve performing the Coccyx Procedure among usual procedures.

BUNIONS

Bunions are caused by a combination of deforming forces. Some are from shoes and stockings, and some are from musculoskeletal dysfunctions. I often pondered why the surgical correction I performed was often impeccable, but the results were less than desired. Many times, the bunion and hallux deformity recurred, months after _successful_ surgery! Most often however, surgery did remain successful. So why, were there a percentage of failures?

Now, I'm convinced that there are two or more major factors. #1. Tight Myofascial leg and foot tissues, #2. Twisting and tilting of the pelvis anatomy.

One of my favorite cases is illustrated by the following:

Chuck's mother, who was a regular patient, asked me if I would see if I could help son's foot problems. One day she said, "Chuck is studying Nursing and he has feet like mine, and I'm afraid he will not be able to stand and walk on concrete floors as required during the normal work shift." When I first saw Chuck, he had all of the foot problems his mother had informed me about. He had bunions, hammertoes, and flat feet. He also had the familiar hip and low back pain that many times follows the unstable feet. I introduced him to my foot rehabilitation and Bowen combination, and after the first week he noted marked improvement. After the second week he returned with improved skin color and a sparkle in his eyes which were not there before. His hygiene and dress was also an 180 Deg. turn. He informed me that he had gotten his first "A" in a test after 2 years of nursing school. He told me how he "crammed for exams, and on the day of the test would kind have choke, and thus "Bees" were about the best he could do. Also, he said, "While I was at my internship last night, I was charting patient notes and all of a sudden I seemed to get everything together." He went on to say," I was afraid that I wasn't going to be a very good nurse because even though I could memorize the material and pass the tests, it didn't make a lot of sense. Now it all has come together." I finished his treatments, made him orthotics, and told him to come back once in a while for a tune-up.

A few weeks later Mildred brought her mother for an appointment. Mildred's Mother didn't speak very fluent English so Mildred told me, "My mother is not eating very well and she has no energy. I know that you are a Foot Doctor, but I want you to give my mother one of those treatments that you do - I go to school with Chuck!" She went on to tell me that about a month ago she noticed a change in Chuck's demeanor. His entire persona had a new character, and she had to ask him what was going on. When he told her that he was having Bowen Therapy and that is all that was different in his life, Mildred concluded that this was responsible in the change in Chuck's life.

Following graduation, I heard via the grapevine that Chuck got 100% on his State Board of Nursing exam. He also has a very good job and has received promotions very quickly. Over the next 2 years Chuck's mother came in every 2 to 3 months for treatment of her corns and calluses. I often asked how Chuck was doing, and she always said that he was, "doing real fine and he was planning to come by for a tune up." One day, he was with his mother during her treatment and we got to talking. I asked," How are your feet doing?" He replied, "Great. My feet have zero pain, and my toes are all straight on the left foot. They are getting straighter on the right foot. At the rate they are changing I think they should all be straight by the year's end." I looked at his mom's feet, which were all deformed with hammertoes and bunions. She'd had "corrective foot surgery" by an orthopedist 4 years before. Her toes were straight for a year or so and then began to re-deform. Something is wrong with this picture. She had surgery and her feet remain deformed. He had no surgery, and his feet are straight. Remember, I hadn't touched this guy for over two years and he's still unwinding!

Now, I can say without any reservation that one can obtain an 80% good result with foot surgery, or you can obtain an 80% or better good results with conservative treatment. This is my conclusion following many similar cases included in my bunion study, in 2004-2005 (which I decided not to publish).

BUNION PROTOCOL

1. Bowen Therapy, complete sessions including; TMJ, Pelvis, all leg muscles and foot intrinsic muscles, once a week for three weeks. See Bunion Procedure.

2. After each session, tape feet as instructed in my photo series.

3. After 3 to 4 weeks, have orthotics made. Do the impressions right after a fresh tape wrap has been done and obtain orthotics or OTC (over-the-counter) supports to maintain foot balance. Pro Lab, Super feet, and Spenco might be the best OTC's. Re-shape and modify as best as possible so they fit flush against the foot which has a *fresh taping applied.*

4. Exercise - Spread the big toe apart from the 2nd toe. Using just the muscle that is supposed to draw the toe toward the mid-line. After a little practice you will be able to do this and you'll feel the Abductor Hallucis muscle under the arch tense up. When you're able to do this, push against the toe with the opposite foot as you perform the exercise. Do this isometric exercise as many times a day as you can, for 2 to 3 minutes each time.

5. Grasp your big toe and stretch in the direction away from the restriction. Maintain the traction for at least 5 minutes. Do both big toes to maintain balance.

6. In addition, use toe spacers @ night and, especially when wearing pantyhose.

7. Be patient and wait and see. It may take months to see results.

8. Get Bowen Tune-ups once a month.

CANCER: In conjunction with her Medical Care

My secretary informed me that a patient was on the phone who needed an appointment for Bowen therapy. She was referred by her neurologist, whom I'd never heard of. Since her only problem was neck pain, my secretary wanted to know if I could see her or not. I said absolutely not, especially since I didn't know the patient nor the referral source. At that point I didn't possess a massage certificate, so I really couldn't wander outside the scope of my Podiatry practice. The next day the lady called back and said, she'd spoken to her neurologist and he insisted that she have Bowen treatments. And, that I was the only person he wanted to touch her. I gave in, and had my receptionist make her an appointment.

When she came for her appointment, we had her sign a waiver that she was fully aware that I was not working as a Podiatrist, but only as a Bowen therapist. As it turned out, she had been going through radiation therapy for breast cancer. She'd had a radical mastectomy with lymph node removal. This had left her with a stiff and painful neck. She was scheduled for a C.T. scan in four weeks to monitor some palpable lymph nodes, so she could only have three weekly treatments. Following which, she would return about a month later for the fourth Bowen treatment after the scan and results were determined, to see if she may need additional surgery for the palpable nodes. After her 1st treatment her range of motion improved about 50%. Following the 2nd treatment her range of motion was about 80 %. After the 3rd session her neck moved pain free in all directions.

When she returned four weeks later she was beaming from ear to ear. Her C.T. scan for the lymph nodes was completely normal. I can't make any conjecture on what transpired other than a spontaneous remission must have occurred. She thought otherwise.

CARPAL TUNNEL

I go for my Zen walk every morning at the nearby botanical garden. I have gotten to know all the employees over time. One morning one of them stopped his golf cart and asked me if I knew anything about carpal tunnel? His main job was mowing acres and acres of grass 4 days a week and the steering of the mower was the probable cause. I told him what I knew, then informed him that I could do a Bowen session. He asked a few questions about Bowen, so as he sat there on his golf cart, I did the Shoulder and Arm Procedures to demonstrate. He felt some immediate changes, then drove off.

I saw him two days later and he told me his hands and wrist were all better. I kept up with him for about 2 years after, until he went to work elsewhere, and he remained pain free.

Most all of the other patients I Treated who had carpal tunnel also resolved. Some recurred due to their repetitive stresses, but again improved with a brief tune-up session.

An interesting side note. My teacher, the late Milton Albrecht, often demonstrated to people with carpal tunnel that by doing the Arm Procedure on the non-symptomatic side-the symptom side would resolve.

CIRCULATION

One December morning a lady came in to get relief for a painful corn on the inner side of her little toe. Her toe was a purplish color with a hard corn on the inner side adjacent to the toenail. She informed me that her toe wasn't always purple. It always got pink when the weather warmed up. She had a condition called Raynaud's disease. Not really a disease, but a spasticity of the blood vessels, which is aggravated by cold temperatures.

She returned in January for another treatment. At this visit she complained about pain in her hip and back due to favoring the pain in her toe. I immediately offered a Bowen session in addition to trimming and padding the corn.

When she returned the following week, her toe was a little less purple and almost pink. I gave her another Bowen treatment, re-padded the corn and advised to come back when necessary.

On a cold, blustery day in February she returned with the painful corn and said," I think that you can go ahead with the operation because the toe has remained pink since the last Bowen treatment." I listened to the pulses with my Doppler ultrasound and sure enough her circulation was totally normal. Her toe was nice and pink, and after I blanched the tip of her toe with finger pressure, it pinked up in 1 second. The following week I operated on the toe and it healed very quickly.

Another patient complained about her cold feet, especially in bed. She had to sleep with her socks on most of the time, and if she didn't her husband complained about her cold feet waking him up all night long. Following 3 treatments her feet warmed up, as well as her hands, and have remained so ever since.

COLDS & FLU

Early in my career as a Bowen therapist a patient was undergoing a session. When I came back into the room following the basic relaxation procedure 3 (neck), she told me that when she got to the office, she was experiencing a severe sore throat. Following the neck muscle releases, the sore throat disappeared. When she returned for another session 2 weeks later, she said," Do you remember that sore throat that I had last time which you cleared?" I replied," yes, what happened?" She told me that when she got home from work that evening her son and husband both had the exact same sore throat and they'd been sick for the past 2 weeks. She didn't get whatever the virus was. I figured that this was some sort of coincidence and went about my business. But other patients told me about similar occurrences. Then, one day I felt the familiar scratchy throat and punky feeling one gets when the cold first comes on. So, I performed the neck moves on myself, and within minutes the symptoms cleared. I've been doing this ever since on myself whenever I feel a cold coming on. I also take a dropper full of Echinacea in a glass of water. It works almost every time. I would only guess that the moves to the neck muscles open up the lymphatic drainage system and this reduces the accumulation of viral bodies in the oral pharynx. Mr. Bowen was notorious for finding the relationship of the lymphatics to the muscles that he moved

COLIC

A young woman came to my office four months after giving birth to a son. She'd gained a lot of weight, and along with the Elastin hormone to give flexibility during the birthing process, her feet collapsed and had become increasingly painful. As I was adhesive taping her feet to lift the arches back up, her 4-month-old baby began to fuss. Her 12-year-old daughter was holding him trying to give comfort. Mom said that he'd had a continuous bout of colic ever since birth and it was quite a strain on everyone. I recalled a couple of Bowen moves that my guru, Milton told me about a few years back and when one of my granddaughters was experiencing colic and it fixed her.

I asked her if it would be okay for me to do a couple gentle movements which might help her. Mom said, "Okay with me." I reached over and moved two muscles across the shoulders twice, and he began to settle a little. I then moved the lower back muscles over the kidneys. And then, did a little arc – like move over the lower abdominal area over the ileum. I showed mom how to do the moves in case she needed to later on if he began to fuss again. He immediately settled down, and his sister fed him a bottle as I performed a Bowen session on the mother.

The next week the mother thanked me for giving her son relief. She didn't need to do any of the moves, because what I did in the office took care of the problem for good. As it turns out, he'd only slept for two hours at a stretch and therefore, so did mom and dad. He also was on medication for projectile vomiting, and didn't any longer require any more medication. He was like a completely new child. He also was unable to nap until the mini treatment session, it was really a mini, and now he naps for two hours at a time. He goes to bed now at around nine o'clock and sleeps straight through until eight AM. Three weeks later, all was still well. As I recall, it only took one session with my granddaughter also.

COCCYX

I received a call recently from a distraught mother of a 15-year-old daughter. She'd had a very painful coccyx for the past 11 months. She had no injury, it just occurred one day. Medications, injections, chiropractic, and physical therapy were all no help. The medical doctor recommended that she have her tailbone surgically removed.

This was quite disturbing to her mom, who is an R.N. at a local Medical Center. A massage classmate of mine recommended that she calls me about Bowen Therapy. The pain was constant, aggravated by arising from a sitting position, and made sleep difficult. She'd been depressed, and had just a plain lousy life the past 11 months as a result.

For those who do Bowen Therapy; I did low back, upper back, neck, lower respiratory, thoraco-lumbar triangle, hamstrings, knee, ankle, pelvis, sacrum, anterior pelvis, coccyx (right to left-right side tender), upper respiratory, TMJ, and my version of cervical release. Her pain began to subside after the coccyx lock on the right side, over the ilio-psoas. When she got off the table, she was pretty much pain-free for the first time in 11 months, and had a big smile on her face. After some tears and hugs, I gave mom a session too. Her mom said when I called her two days later, that about 50% of the pain was gone, but anti-inflammatory medication got her pain free. Previously it did not. The next week mom told me that the pain had returned a little as the day of treatment wore on, but she did get a good night's sleep. Following her 2nd and 3rd visits she remains pain free.

DEPRESSION

As I performed a Bowen session on a woman one afternoon, we got talking and I told her the story about Chuck, the nursing student, and how his personality blossomed after two therapy sessions. She asked, "Would you please give my 13-year-old son some treatments? He's been very angry and withdrawn ever since my divorce." I told her I could, and to go ahead, and make an appointment for him. On his first visit, he didn't say three words. He barely answered the couple of questions I asked him. I didn't pay any mind to the fact that he was wearing entirely black clothing. Following the session, I said goodbye to he and his mother as they made his next appointment. The following week he seemed a little more conversive as I made small talk. During one of the rest periods, I went out to the waiting room and asked mom how the week went. She said," Allen has really perked up. His anger is less, and he's wearing other colored clothing besides all black." When I went back into the treatment room, I saw that he was wearing a bright, yellow T-shirt with black shorts. As the weeks passed, he became more outgoing, friendly, and became socially active again according to his mother. His next appointment he had made for himself. And, he looked forward to more follow up sessions in the months to follow.

DIGESTIVE DISORDERS

Over the years, (1995 - 2012) I've had a good number of patients with; Irritable Bowel Syndrome, Diarrhea, Constipation, Gallbladder, Colic issues improve or resolve. I've done many sessions for patients at a local oncology Clinic who were suffering from the side effects of chemotherapy. As long as they came regularly, their pain and nausea are controlled.

FIBROMYALGIA

When I incorporated Bowen Therapy into my podiatry practice the patients who had a diagnosis of fibromyalgia either did very well, or not. I soon came to some conclusions:

That some patients think they have FM because their doctor told them but don't really have it. Others who do have FM, have varying degrees of severity. Because it affects mostly women and rarely men, it is my belief that there must be some hormonal element to it.

I learned to do the following when a patient tells me they have FM. If a massage is agreeable and feels good, Bowen will likely help. If a massage is painful during or after – Bowen will likely be painful too. If they are opposed to massage, try Bowen to see if it helps them. If a little bit is good then proceed from there. Use the CHAIRSIDE REBOOT, found on page 8.

For those who experience too much pain from massage and Bowen, John F. Barnes's, "MYOFASCIAL RELEASE" technique, is very good.

OPTIONAL PROCEDURE FOR INTENSE PAIN

Milton, my instructor, first taught me this procedure during one of our fireside chats circa 2000. He explained, "Use this when your client is in so much pain that they can't get up on the table. It will relax them so they can move a little better, and then they can get up on the table." I found this procedure helpful for patients who were in acute spasms. It enabled them to be slightly more mobile, and it only took a minute or so to do.

K.C., who was one of my long time, regular patients said, "I met your guru, Uncle Milty. I went to his house with a friend and he cleared up my gallbladder problem. Just to think that I was going to have surgery for my gallbladder, and now I won't!" I was happy for her and we talked a bit about Milton and Bowen during the rest of her podiatry visit that morning.

K.C. came in for her podiatry appointment. She lamented, "Oh, I sure wish our Uncle Milty was still here. My gallbladder problem has resurfaced, and my doctor wants me to have surgery. I'm having a second opinion tomorrow. I remember how Milton fixed my problem, and that was over 4 years ago." I offered, "I can give you a Bowen session."

I overheard my nurse bringing her into one of my Bowen rooms and she said, "This is your first Bowen with Dr. Mosher isn't it? You need to take your shoes off and lay face down on the table with your feet on the pillow and your face in the face cradle." K.C. replied, "Oh no. I don't have to lie down for this. we can just do it standing up." I realized what she was referring to so, I quickly stepped in to save an argument. I said, "You mean to tell me that all Milton did for you that time you saw him was the standing procedure?" She replied, "That's right. He did it right there in his living room and I was fine all those years." So, I did the standing Optional Procedure for her, and she has been fine ever since.

At massage school I performed this procedure on a number of classmates with equally good results. FM is mostly associated with chemicals, free radicals, and toxins. Since the condition has increased in its frequency since the 1980's. Our exposure to chemicals in foods, beverages, personal care and cleaning products, and oil-based pesticides has risen also. Consumption of poultry and meats provide us with doses of antibiotics continually. These upset our normal bacteria flora in the gut, so digestion becomes impaired. 70% of the immune system comes from the gut and the digestion issue compromises it. Poorly digested foods also turn toxic.

Muscles are fatigued and lacking ATP, build up lactic acid, stay contracted. CoQ10 is needed for muscle function. That's why patients develop muscle pains when taking statin drugs, as they deplete the CoQ10 levels.

FM is often associated with chronic fatigue syndrome. Compromised immune system is associated with both FM and CFS.

HEEL PAIN / PLANTAR FASCIITIS

Plantar fasciitis (fash-ee-itis, often pronounced face-ee-it is), is one of those medical enigmas (mysteries). It is one of the most intriguing to me of all of the foot maladies I encountered. I consider myself an expert on PF since I've been a health care provider and educator for over 40 years, and I've treated and helped thousands of patients during those years.

At one point, I had quite a few heavier women who came to me with pain in their heel/heels. They were usually around _45 to 65_ years old. They mostly wore flip-flops or backless shoes. They had severe pain when arising that subsided after 15 - 20 minutes of ambulation. There was an occasional man who fit the same model. X-Rays usually showed a heel spur, but not always, (this is significant for this problem - plus many other pain issues). Other male and female overweight patients came in with the same story, however the X-rays did not show a heel spur. I found spurs on thousands of X-Rays and the patient never had any associated pain. At one time there was a chiropractic study done on 100 subjects who had zero history of back pain. After MRI's were performed on them, 40% had bulging disks.

As years went by, lots of younger women and men, without excess weight, came in to see me with the same symptoms. Some had spurs on their X-ray's, others didn't.

I was baffled. Cortisone shot helped one, but not the other. Orthotics helped one, but not the other. Surgical removal of the spur was a miracle for one, but made the next one worse. I even employed the use of an ultrasound imagery device which showed exactly where I was placing the needle, and the cortisone injection. This helped a little, but not a miracle. Physical Therapy hardly ever worked. Acupuncture & Chiropractic did not always help either.

When I performed ultrasounds on my PF patients the fascia was most always thickened with a swollen area below it. I always did bilateral images. The non-symptom side was never swollen. Often, a patient would return a year or two later with pain in the other heel. Ultrasound images showed that the previous heel was still thickened and swollen, even though it had been pain free for the past year or two. One thing I did observe was that I never saw a patient with PF who wore cowboy boots or solid dress shoes. Every one wore soft, walking, or running shoes.

Heel pain may be a result of the following:

- Inflammation of the fascia.
- Inflammation of the periosteum.
- Stress fracture.
- Strain of Flexor Brevis and or Quadratus Plantae muscles.
- Subluxation of the Calcaneal - Cuboid joint.
- Shortening of the Gastrocnemius Muscle (Calf Muscle).
- Compression of the Sciatic Nerve.

So, x-rays, ultrasound, MRI, nuclear bone scans can all be helpful in the diagnosis and treatment of heel pain. Obviously, if one has a sciatic nerve problem a steroid injection in the plantar fascia is not going to help.

However, after I learned how to perform Bowen's Therapy in 1995, a little more light was shed on the subject. Tightened lower leg muscles which were released, offered another solution. Release of the Gluteal and Piriformis muscles over the sciatic nerve offered some others a solution.

Walla- Stretching. The missing piece to the plantar fasciitis puzzle.

My last year in practice, I began prescribing a DynaSplint ® device. This splint holds the foot and ankle at a position of stretch which decompresses the blood vessels so they can dilate and allow more blood flow in, and also lets the stagnate blood flow out - not rocket science. My patients had to comply for 5 hours, (cumulatively), per day. Those that did, it was a miracle. Those that did not were so-so.

OTHER OPTIONS:

1. Get a 3-foot heavy, black rubber, bungee cord. Place it under the ball of your foot and pull back with your hands. Increase the pressure and push your foot down against the resistance. Do both feet so there isn't an imbalance. Stretch for 3 to 5 minutes per foot as many times a day as you can.

2. Stretch as in #1, before you get out of bed in the morning.

3. Put your shoes on, and lace them up, before you hit the floor in the morning. This gives your foot some protection. While sleeping, your body is in the healing mode. When you arise, you can undo what has been heeling the past 8 hours, so - be careful! Do not walk without your best shoes on. Wear the same shoes that offer the most comfort.

4. Add ¼ - ½ inch heel lifts, wear wedgies, or cowboy boots.

5. While sitting at your computer, roll your foot - heel and arch over a golf ball. Do both feet.

6. Stretch your calf muscles for 3 to 5 minutes. Lean against a wall and push your pelvis toward the wall which will place a stretch on the calf muscles.

7. Purchase over the counter arch supports such as Super Feet, or Spenco. The Spencos can be heated and re-shaped to fit the contour of the arch.

8. Tape your arches. - See video: http://www.youtube.com/channel/UCd8pRsoyYXLy3rPNKgbk6IQ?feature=results_main

9. Have your partner hold onto your heels and lean back while you are lying on your back. This will stretch your fascia from head to toe. Do for a minimum of 3 to 5 minutes.

10. Replace any shoes that the heels are worn down on the outer side.

Health Maintenance Options from A to Z for Plantar Fasciitis

- Acupuncture.
- Bowen - Get 3 Bowen Therapy sessions a week apart. Video: https://www.youtube.com/channel/UCd8pRsoyYXLy3rPNKgbk6IQ
- Cam Walker.
- Chiropractic. Find a podiatrist or chiropractor who does foot manipulations. Activators ® work wonders.
- Cortisone injection.
- Dyna Splint.
- Homeopathy.
- Joint mobilization and manipulation.
- MENS - electrical stimulation. MENS micro current therapy aids in cell stimulation for healing.
- MFR Myofascial Release and Cranio Sacral therapies.
- NSAID'S.
- Orthotics.
- Podiatrist. Find a podiatrist who; has an in-house ultrasound, will place a TENS unit in proximity to the heel to reduce injection pain, place local anesthetic around the Calcaneal Nerve, before injecting the cortisone, and guides the needle into the appropriate spot with ultrasound visualization.
- Surgery, Plantar fascia release. My surgery of choice was the per-cutaneous technique when all else failed. It is the least invasive of the surgical procedures. Recovery time is much shorter and complications are rare. I only had one mishap out of hundreds of procedures I performed with that technique.
- Tape strapping. Find a podiatrist who will strap your arch - I will provide a tutorial on how to do so on YouTube. And then, get some orthotics, once your pain has subsided.

Case study:

One of my patients, who I had treated off and on for about 3 years for plantar fasciitis, came in for her semi-annual cortisone injection. I had tried everything except surgery and Bowen. When I informed her about Bowen, and that there was a chance it could relieve her pain, she quickly agreed to it. This was about 2 months after I had taken my 1st Bowen workshop in 1995.

Lorna was a very large lady, about 260 pounds. Muscle mass was very large and taut, beneath adipose tissue. She was wearing a dress, which inhibited my doing the pelvis and hamstrings procedures properly, so, I did what I could. I performed BRP 1, BRP, 2, BRP 3, aka BRM's, KIDNEY, LOWER RESPIRATORY, HAMSTRINGS, ANTERIOR PELVIS, KNEE, ANKLE, UPPER RESPIRATORY, AND TMJ. When I finished, I said, "Rest for a couple minutes, the get up and walk around a minute or two before you put your shoes back on. I will see you before you leave". While I was with another patient, I heard a yell, "Yahoo!" I rushed in and asked, "Is everything was okay?" She said, "Yeah. I got up to walk over to your desk to get my glasses and the pain is completely gone. Wow!"

We hired Lorna shortly after to clean our offices once a week. When I retired in 2006, she was still pain free. I never treated her one time with any modality since that day in 1995.

INFERTILITY

Fertility issues appear to be focused on the brain-pituitary-ovarian axis among some other events. Stress, negative emotions, and unbalanced FSH disrupt the hormonal communication between the brain, pituitary, and ovaries. Sympathetic overdrive decreases ovarian blood flow and egg production as well.

PCOS = Polycystic Ovary Syndrome is a contributor of infertility.

"We've recently demonstrated that women with PCOS have a highly active sympathetic nervous system, the part that isn't controlled by our will, and that both acupuncture and regular exercise reduced levels of activity in this system compared with the control group, which could be an explanation for the results," said Stener-Victorin.

High levels of FSH in women is a signal of a loss of, or poor ovarian function, polycystic ovary syndrome or can indicate that menopause has begun, or is currently taking place. All of these conditions will have a negative impact on fertility. Low levels of FSH can indicate that eggs are not being produced, that the pituitary gland is not functioning correctly, that there are significant levels of stress present, or that the person is severely underweight which is causing problems to occur.

Acupuncture appears to have an effect on hormonal balancing. Production and release of beta endorphin and peptides into the central and peripheral nervous systems; reduces anxiety and stress, improves sleep, decreases or increases levels of FSH, decreases sympathetic overdrive, increases ovarian and uterine blood flow which aids in endometrial thickness, increased follicles and egg production.

Candace Pert, Ph.D., points out that her research found; high concentrations of beta endorphin in the node points along the spine, and that beta endorphin mediates communication between the central, immune, and endocrine systems.

Other research using fine needle biopsies of the meridian node points and fluid analysis reveals peptides, beta endorphin, and many other bio-chemicals from these points. Guess where these points are located? Along the Bladder and Governing Vessel Meridians, adjacent to the spine. Exactly where Tom's BRM moves are placed.

It was not surprising that many of my patients who had fertility issues became pregnant following one to three Bowen sessions. One had only zero to 2 unusable eggs per cycle for IVF during the past 8 months. A week after her second Bowen session, she produced 28 eggs!

Case study: This paper addresses only the female issues of infertility.

When this subject came for Bowen, I was skeptical if Bowen would help. But when I questioned Milton about it later, he casually remarked, "That Bowen Therapy straightened the fallopian tubes so the eggs can drop, and thus become impregnated when the timing is right. When the tube is bent because the posture alignment is bent, the eggs can't drop." About two years later, three of my patients miraculously became pregnant following Bowen Therapy. They came in about one month apart. The first patient came specifically for that purpose as she had read in a magazine publication that Bowen Therapy was successful with infertility issues. The other two had mentioned their infertility problems, but I never said anything to them about Bowen Therapy helping infertility. I found out later that they all recently gotten pregnant.

Marcy, one of my podiatry patients, had been favoring her foot pain during the past few weeks, which made her back painful. In addition to caring for her foot pain, I gave her two Bowen sessions a week apart. I did my usual routine, plus what she needed for her back pain. When she returned the third week she was grinning from ear to ear. She said, "Thank you." I said, "Thank me for what? You don't have to thank me for fixing your foot." She replied, "I've been going to the infertility clinic during the past eight months. Every month, I only produce one or two eggs, if that, and none have been satisfactory for insemination. Last week, I had twenty eight eggs! They harvested three and put twelve in my egg bank."

Eight months later she had twins. She's convinced that the Bowen Therapy was responsible for this.

One morning I met up with the acupuncturist, who practiced next door to me, out in the parking lot. I asked, "How exactly, does acupuncture help infertility?" He replied. "Studies have shown that the stimulation of the meridians and meridian points causes stimulation of the hypothalamus which affects the pituitary gland, which causes the production of gonadotropic hormones, which then stimulates increased sperm and egg production."

This acupuncturist was one of my first people to practice Bowen on right after I learned it. After his first session for a knee problem, he said, "Wow! That's as close to acupuncture as I've ever experienced, only without the needles!" Considering that many of the Bowen moves are over significant meridian points and over the tissues where the meridian ductules have to pass through, it's distinctly possible that a similar effect as acupuncture takes place, which results in increased egg production.

BOWEN PROCEDURES AND PROTOCOL:

BRMS: Low back, Upper back & shoulder, Neck, Lumbar aka Kidney, Para spinal Itsy- Bitsy's from S-1 to C-1, coccyx, and anterior pelvis with lots of long rests. Total session time = 60 minutes. Another Bowen session, five to seven days before ovulation using the same format. And, remember the word, "Intent."

MIGRAINES

Quite often patients will experience a flare of present symptoms. Kind of, like when one has a fever, the fever spikes just before it subsides for good. Other times old, pains come out of the closet. There can be a reoccurrence of an old problem, which has seemingly been resolved for a number of months or years? These unpleasant reactions usually don't last more than a few hours or a day. This is called a, "Herxheimer's reaction".

One of my patients experienced the following incredible sequence. At the completion of Traci's first therapy session, I explained the above to her. When she returned the following week she said, "You won't believe what happened. When I got home the day of the treatment, my T.M.J. flared up for about six hours. That night I got a throbbing headache, which was gone by morning. Then my neck tightened up until noontime. Then my shoulder froze up until dinner, and then everything's been fine ever since. I've been totally pain free all week." I replied, "That isn't too unusual." She said, "You don't understand. That's the exact sequence that these problems began to surface five years ago. I had a bout with my T.M.J. for about a year. Then I began experiencing headaches two to three times a week. A year later, my neck tightened and would spasm once or twice a month. Then, a year ago my shoulder froze up and has been painful to lift my arm much higher than my waist." As the weeks went by during her postural and foot realignment process these symptoms didn't return. Traci moved to the East Coast shortly after. Her mother-in-law came to me on occasion for Bowen sessions, so I always asked her how Traci was doing with regard to all of her aches and pains? She said, "Traci says thanks. She's not had any pain at all this past year since she moved."

NECK PAIN

The most dramatic case of neck pain was a patient I treated early in my Bowen Therapy learning process. I met a massage therapist who had a chronic neck issue. She'd never heard of the Bowen technique, but wanted to see what it was all about. After a single session her neck problem resolved. She was so impressed with the simplicity of the technique and the power of its results; she took my class. She is now a very proficient Bowen practitioner.

PARKINSON'S

One patient indicated that by her last visit, her tremors were reduced by 70 to 80%. A few others had improvement with their pains, but not much with their tremors. In the cases of another patient, is virtually pain free, reducing her medication week to week, and about to abandon her cane. Her foot is straighter also. One other has much less pain, more strength, and ambulates better. Her feet remain rigid and misaligned.

SCIATICA

When I got to the office on the first Monday morning after my Bowen class, the very first patient needed the treatment. She had a sciatic nerve problem in the past and she was certain that it had reoccurred because she had been performing floor exercises for long periods of time and now her left foot had a tingling sensation like the previous bout with sciatica.

I informed her about the new therapy I'd just learned and offered it to her. It took less than a nanosecond for her to say yes. I escorted her into my operating room which I had transformed into a temporary therapy room and placed her on the surgical gurney which I'd converted into a temporary massage table. I quickly checked my notes from the seminar and began the treatment. I only performed the treatment in the waist, legs, and feet to stay within the boundaries of my Podiatry license. When the session ended, she got up and stood on her feet she said, "'It sure feels better. Not all the way but at least 50%".

The next morning, she called me to report, "That by noon Monday all of the symptoms had disappeared, and the next time she got the sciatica back she would call me for treatment."

Since then, I've used the sciatic #1 and Sciatic #2 Bowen procedures on hundreds of patients and it works almost every time. And, most of the time the relief is permanent.

SHOULDER

One Sunday afternoon, I dropped in on one of my guru's Basic Bowen classes. Milton was starting on the Frozen Shoulder procedure as I got in the room.

His opening story goes like -- One of his buddies called him one Sunday morning and begged him to help with his frozen shoulder. Milt said, "It's my day off, so call me tomorrow." And hung up on him. An hour later, the doorbell rang, and when Milton opened the door there was his buddy. He showed Milton how he couldn't raise his arm. He told Milt about how he had all these chores to do, but couldn't because of the shoulder. Milt invited him into the living room and asked, "Which shoulder hurts?" The buddy said, "The right one."

Milton had him turn sideways so his left shoulder was facing him. Milton then struck the buddies left shoulder with his fist about as hard as he could. The blow about knocked the guy across the room. The buddy said, "Hey. What'd you do?" Milt said, "Shut up. I just fixed your shoulder." The buddy said, "You made my good arm hurt?" Milt said, " That's okay. Try it out." Buddy raised his arm on the bad shoulder side and it was all loosened and the pain was gone.

I went home and did the same procedure on my wife (Not a Bowen Procedure). She'd had shoulder pain for over six months. Guess what? Monday morning her pain was all gone, and has never returned.

There is a Frozen Shoulder Bowen procedure that is highly effective to relieve shoulder pain and tightness.

SINUSES

One Friday afternoon after I'd completed the same neck moves on a patient, she commented that her sinus infection cleared up while I was out of the room. I commented something or another, and then she asked, "If my husband can get here before closing time, could you give him a treatment too? He has the same sinus infection that I had."

TMJ

When I had my first Bowen session, my TMJ was shifting to the right. I was constantly nipping my cheek while chewing my food. Milton had me place a finger between my teeth, then performed some movements to the muscles around my jaw. After I removed the finger and opened my jaw, it was perfect alignment.

TENNIS ELBOW

One of my first few Bowen patients came to me with Tennis Elbow. She was seeded number 1 in her age group at a local tennis club. She dropped to fourth due to the fact that she couldn't serve as well as needed. This riled her enormously as she was a feisty, competitive, 60-year-old. One session was all it took, and she quickly went back to # 1. At last count, she had referred me 36 new patients that I was aware of!

Recently, I treated a young lady who had severe symptoms for over six months. She even had to hold her drinking glass in her other hand. After I performed the Shoulder and Arm Procedures, she could feel immediate changes taking place. The next day her mother left a lengthy voice mail telling me that her daughter was completely pain free.

TRAUMA

Ethyl was referred to me by her chiropractor. She was hit by a car 9 years before we met and suffered major trauma to her right leg and foot. Following multiple surgeries and rehabilitation, she was stuck on morphine and other narcotics, until one day she decided to get off the drugs. Then, her back and foot became more painful, so her chiropractor wanted me to make orthotics for her feet with hopes that her back would stay in longer following adjustment. She walked with a noticeable limp, she was unable to rise up on her toes and she had a mass of scarring in the lower leg. She spoke very rapidly with a slight stammer, and seemed quite hyper. On her initial visit I gave her an abbreviated Bowen session due to time constraints, and taped her arch for temporary support. She noted immediate improvement in her foot as well as her back pain.

The following week she was a lot better and was looking forward to a full Bowen treatment, which I did. When she returned the following week, I saw her standing in the waiting room near the hall door, and I asked her, "How are you doing?" She smiled and motioned with her index finger to come here. As I crossed the threshold, she put out her arms and gave me one of those 'Warm fuzzy hugs' and whispered in my ear, "Thank you. I'm a brand-new person. I can get up on my toes, my foot doesn't hurt, and my back is 80% better. I worked in my vegetable garden for hours without getting tired and sore. And, everyone at work noticed that I'm walking normally now."

Another case that I was involved with early on in my Bowen Therapy career came to light two years hence. Big John came to my office for his initial visit. He said, "I need one of those Bowen treatments you do. My friend Peter says they are a miracle. You fixed his back pain with one treatment and my back is killing me, so can you fix me too."

When I returned to the room after the customary 3-minute rest between moves to the muscles, He said, "I remember Peter's last name mate, it's Hubbard." After I completed the next series of moves, I went to the chart files and pulled Peter Hubbard's chart. When I glanced at my chart notes I remembered the Patient and the incident. Peter had been in a car-motorcycle accident at age sixteen. His right ankle had been badly fractured. He had many surgical procedures, 2 years of physical therapy, a set of custom foot orthotics, and done home therapy exercises over the years. He was told at age nineteen it would not improve anymore and he was stuck with a permanent clubfoot deformity and posttraumatic arthritis.

On the day of Peter's 1st visit he told me his story, and was concerned about his orthotics not fitting properly as he had them for many years. His leg muscle was in spasm, and he was walking differently due to these problems. I do not remember, nor did I note in the chart anything about back pain. But it is very frequent that when one favors a foot deformity or pain, they will experience back pain. I gave Peter a Bowen treatment for the muscle spasm and the other postural pains he was experiencing. I kept his orthotics for a week in order to refurbish them, and he came for a second appointment a week later. I gave him a second Bowen treatment, placed the orthotics in his shoe and reappointed him for one week for a follow up visit which he failed to keep. When I finished looking at his chart my curiosity got the best of me and I walked out of my office to the parking lot and saw him sitting in the passenger seat reading a book. I said, "Hi Peter. Thanks for bringing Big John for a treatment. What is going on?" He looked up and replied, "Oh, Dr. Mosher! I'm sorry I never came back to thank you for taking care of me. I know that you're very busy and I didn't want to bother you and I am lousy at writing letters." I inquired as to what had transpired and he told me the following.

He didn't return for the follow up visit because he didn't notice any difference in the symptoms and pain he was experiencing. However, 4 weeks after the treatments, while retiring to bed one night his ankle started to itch quite badly. Not in the skin, but, "way down deep". It had kept him awake for a couple of hours, and the subsided enough for him to dose off. During the night the itching would wake him up, but then he would go back to a light sleep. When he got up the next morning his foot and ankle were noticeably more limber, and slightly less painful.

The same thing happened 4 weeks later, and 4 weeks after that. He said that, "About every 4 weeks for about 14 months his foot would itch at bedtime for one night only, and each time he noticed better range of motion and lessened pain upon arising the next morning. Presently, he had no further foot deformity, no leg muscle spasms, and no more back pain." I have seen Peter off and on over the years for minor "Tune-ups" and he remains just fine with regards to his ankle. He recalled on one occasion that when he told me that afternoon at my office that he was all better, he really was only about 90% better. It took another year to a year and a half to get all the way well. Also in is interesting that the majority of his recovery took 14 months since he was 14 years post injury. That's 1 month for every year, interesting observation.

THE MILTON ALBRECHT CONNECTION & THE BOWEN TECHNIQUE

I am putting this paper together because the late Milton Albrecht changed; my life, podiatry career, retirement, and many of my patient's lives. Milton also has directly and indirectly enhanced the legacy and training of the Bowen Technique worldwide, and this may be unbeknownst to many Bowen practitioners. He may also have had some direct or indirect influence on your training or career even though you had never personally met him. But, BTW - you may have already met him - via me or maybe someone else?

This tribute is to create more awareness of this great man who figured out many of our "Advanced or Special" Procedures, trained many of the present-day practitioners, instructors, and then left some of his lore prior to passing in 2003.

My first encounter with Milton was in October 1994. He was always a very enthusiastic mentor for me as well as with many of his other students and associates.

My attempts to obtain more input from Milt's students and clients to add to this paper so far have fallen a little short, so the recounting of Milton and his Bowen involvement is my recall, a few other's stories including his late wife Denis' tribute, and one of his closest friends who teaches in Milt's shadow. I am hoping for some more input from; his sister Debbie, his students, and some of his patient 's folklore about Milt. He was quite a character while at the same time a very powerful ambassador of Bowen Therapy as you will discover.

It has been documented that Tom Bowen acknowledged only 6 men in his fold prior to his passing in 1982. They were called "Tom's Boys" by his receptionist Renee Horwood. In 1989 one of the men showed the late Milton Albrecht how to perform his "Interpretation of Tom Bowen's Technique. If Tom had lived to know Milton, he likely would have acknowledged him too, as Milt was a master at "Working it out."

PAINTING A PICTURE OF THE LATE MILTON ALBRECHT

This was a Bowen Therapist and Teacher that you need to know about

I bet Milton was a hellion in high school. He had traumatic arthritis in one of his ankles that resulted from a fracture when he was attacked by a SOB at a drive-in parking lot.

His occupation Before Bowen (B.B) was a machinist / mechanic. He built race car engines and hot rods. So, he had great tactile and common senses. He put these to use in his Bowen career. He also seemed to develop a 6th sense over the years that I knew him. He became a "medical intuitive" so to speak.

Whenever the legal people came to him for a copy of his medical records his reply was, "I don't keep any records. It's all in my head. You can keep your $5.00. I can't give you a copy of any records."

When doctors called him for information, he often hung up on them. Milt had a profound distrust of most doctors. He trusted; me, a local oncologist, the late doctor Joanne Whitaker, and some of his doctor Bowen students from around the world. Sorry if I left anyone out.

At a party or social gathering he would often do some moves on the side opposite of the problem and clear up the problem (next Monday - surgery cancelled).

He often treated people in his living room, back patio, or front porch besides in his massage tables set up in two of his bedrooms.

His usual daily dress code was Bermuda shorts, half buttoned shirt, bare foot, shave maybe, and hair might be combed, or maybe not.

Milt's usual Bowen session was a mish mosh of the 23 procedures that Bowtech outlined in their 14 pages of "The Notes". Circa 1990's. However, I noticed over the years he followed certain patterns. So did his cousin Albert, and one of his assistants Joan. That's where my recipe sequence came from. (See the files sections in; Bowen Therapy Worldwide, Bowen Therapy USA, and Bowen Therapy Education Worldwide). He also added in extra procedures when they were needed (many of which he eventually called DTO's (Don't tell Ossie). This is explained in his wife Deni's Tribute to Milton.)

Milt also performed the more is better technique – lots of procedures most of the time on most of his clients. His reason was, "When someone takes time off work and drives an hour to come see you - they deserve a full session." Milt knew that Tom only spent about 5 to 7 minutes with his clients. Otherwise, how could Tom possibly see 65 to 70 clients a day whilst doing a full body session?

He had an unlisted phone number, no sign on the street, no listing in the phone book, only answered his phone between 8:00 AM and 9:00 AM, and did not return calls left on his answering machine / voice mail.

He treated 25 to 30 people a day except when the flu season hit or the weather was bad. When I made my first appointment, he was booked out for three weeks. He could have seen more clients a day except he was busy taking care of his invalid wife Deni, doing some internet stuff, and working on his classes.

His feet were in poor condition (he rarely wore footwear). I went to his house after patients every couple of months to trim his calluses and get a Bowen Tune-up for myself, along with some of his words of wisdom. I wish that I had taken notes when I was there L. He told me a lot of stuff that I don't remember. He told me lots more than I do recall and I will pass that on to you later. One thing he often related to me was that he could feel Tom's presence and guidance while he was working it out on a client.

Milt also had a keen command of the four-letter word vocabulary.

Milt always dressed up for his Bowen Classes. Face shaved, hair combed, long pants, shirt buttoned up and Van's slip-on shoes with no socks.

He preferred to teach people who had no massage, chiropractic, or medical background. He found the lay public more coachable. Believe it or not some very proficient Bowen Practitioners came from that demographic. In my class the massage therapists caught on to it much quicker than the rest of us. His classes were usually about 25 to 30 students. He usually started a class by saying, "I'm not a teacher but I'm going to show all of you this Bowen Technique which might change some of your lives."

I often admonished Milt to quit smoking. His reply was always, "The three loves of my life are taking care of my wife, doing Bowen Therapy, and smoking a cigarette. I will never give up on any of them."

Milt passed over at about 3:00 AM on the morning of January 14, 2003 at the tender age of 53.

I know that Milton still watches after me while I "work it out" on my patients and show it to my students. He always has and always will.

Following is what one of our colleagues and instructor says about Milton:

I want to offer a huge "thank you" to Mitchell Mosher for his moving tribute to the late Milton Albrecht, the founder of Bowen Therapy International following the sad events causing the big breakaway split with Bowtech back in 1997 when many of us were left in the wind. Milton was so special in our hearts, and his lovely wife Deni and I became extra special friends after his untimely passing in 2003. She and I were extremely close allies in our quest to protect and promote Milton's passion, his interpretation and dedication to Tom Bowen's work. For the past 12 years, as Bowen partners-in-crime, sometimes against all odds, we tried to stay true in honor of both Mr. Bowen and Milton - who I am sure Tom would have considered to be 'The 7th Man" had they had the good fortune to meet. I will never forget Milton or Deni and will strive to honor their passion for this amazing gift that we in the Bowen world have been fortunate to share with those who may benefit from it. This is truly a gift of love that has been passed down through a grateful band of blessed recipients, and I, for one, will never forget Milton who holds a special place in our hearts. We will continue to fly the Bowen flag as this work is too important not to get the recognition it deserves. A big "thank you" to Milt, Deni, Julian Baker (who made it all possible for us in the first place), and all our other Bowen friends out there! Cheryll

About Milton Albrecht

Before Milt became a Bowen Therapist he had a machine shop, built race car engines, and hot rods. He was born, raised, and lived his entire life in and around Auburn, California, a foothills town on the way to the Sierra mountains and Lake Tahoe. He knew most everyone in town except the recent transplants.

Milt married a childhood acquaintance, Deni Larrimore, and she was instrumental in bringing Bowen Therapy to the US in 1989. Deni had suffered cervical pain in early adulthood after the local G.P.'s gave her some cortisone injections in her neck. Sometime later she developed signs of MS and then experienced continual back pain. Milton was convinced that the cortisone injections were what led to her symptoms. At this point she was managing the pain with pain medications. Until, Milt learned the Bowen Technique!

Milton's late wife Deni Larimore Albrecht wrote the following Tribute to "Milt", as he was often referred to. This is posted on The Parker School of Bowenology website.

Milton J. Albrecht, First Bowen U.S. Pioneer

Milton J. Albrecht, the first Bowen Therapist and instructor certified in North America 1948-2003
Milton J. Albrecht was the first Bowen therapist certified outside of Australia, sponsoring the first Bowen seminar held in the U.S., in September, 1989. Becoming internationally well-known for his progressive interpretation of Tom Bowen's Australian modality.

Milton Joseph Albrecht – A loving tribute by Deni Larimore Albrecht

Born on November 12, 1948, Milton was a lifelong resident of Auburn, California. He had already established a career as a highly regarded automotive machinist, when he and I married in April, 1985. Milton and I were first briefly introduced when I was around 13, but had no connection for the next 15 years. When we met again in September, 1984, I was confined to a wheelchair due to a diagnosis of multiple sclerosis, 11 years earlier.

On a solo trip to visit my parents in Sydney, Australia, in January, 1989, I had my first two Bowen treatments from Ossie Rentch (a student of Tom Bowen). Ossie and his wife Elaine were sheep ranchers in Victoria, who had known my folks for years, and Mother & Dad felt sure he could help me. A few months later, Ossie flew to San Francisco to organize his first North American Bowen training seminars, and Milton met him at the airport. Spending the first night at our house, Ossie briefly taught Milton the fundamentals of Bowen, because I had been noticing improvements from those first treatments in January. September 10-12, 1989, Milton and I sponsored the first Bowen seminar held outside of Australia/New Zealand, and Milton earned the first Bowen therapy diploma in North America. Although he took the class primarily to help me, the Rentsch's were so impressed with his natural abilities and talent, they suggested Milton become a full-time Bowen therapist. Because he was already quite enthusiastic, Milton took the step that would change not only his life, but the lives of thousands. We were also asked to coordinate Ossie's organization, Bowtech, here in North America, and in addition, began the first weekly student practice sessions, which we continued in our home for many years.

Milton worked very hard to promote Bowen, and treated everyone he could, friends and family alike. To add state legitimacy, he quickly enrolled in a general massage course, to earn a certificate in massage therapy (CMT). The instructors raved about his bodywork abilities, but Milton continually promoted Bowen, and demonstrated it at every juncture possible. He even secretly used Bowen during the final practical exam, and his instructor proclaimed it the best "massage" he had ever experienced.

Because of his mechanical background, Milton understood the body worked like a machine, and applied this understanding to each client he worked with. His granddaughter was born with a severe clubfoot, and after just one Bowen session, it began correcting itself ! Doctors were astounded as she had been scheduled for corrective surgery, and today, that baby is a 17-year-old flyer on her high school cheerleading team. One of Milton's uncles was experiencing chest pain and difficulty breathing, and Milton used Bowen to bring about immediate relief. A few years later, this procedure (Bowen therapists call these "moves") came to the attention of renowned cardiologists in San Francisco, who contacted Milton about the drastic improvements they were noticing in mutual patients. (Students came to know this as the "Uncle Frank"

Milton's passion for Bowen constantly overflowed, and he could not wait to show Ossie his new developments. Ossie would always remark, "well, is it Bowen?", and of course, the answer was always yes. At that time, Bowtech had only two courses, beginning and certification, and the Rentch's traveled to North America once or twice a year, to conduct courses in several regions of the US and Canada. In September, 1992, for an article about Tom Bowen, Ossie was interviewed by Massage Magazine. But he couldn't make the photo shoot, so the sidebar included pictures of Milton using Bowen with a very willing reporter. (I was asked to write the description.)

Due to Milton's popularity, Auburn classes were always full. So realizing even further Milton's genius, in 1994, Ossie asked Milton to teach beginning Bowtech classes. As he became the first Bowen instructor not taught directly by Tom Bowen, delighted clients flocked to Milton's classes. In addition, Milton traveled throughout the US with the Rentschs, and at seminar venues, alternative medical conventions, and even the prestigious HeartMath at Stanford, Milton demonstrated the effectiveness of Bowen therapy, as Ossie lectured. In one particular case, Milton used Bowen therapy to turn a breach baby in the womb. (To everyone's surprise, except Milton, the baby was later delivered without complications!).

By this time, Milton's clientele was huge, and 60% of his clients were new, each day! As was the case with Tom Bowen, Milton never advertised, and even though he saw 25 people a day, six days a week, his reputation grew strictly by word of mouth. He usually saw 4 people each hour, and because there are usually 2-10 minute waiting periods between moves, Milton could go from client to client. He would often ask the client's family or friends to observe the session so he could explain not only what he was doing, but how they could help themselves in the future. Milt (as I called him) was interviewed several times by Cary Nosler (Captain Carrot) on his healthy living radio program, and demonstrated Bowen to the San Francisco 49er football head trainer, who unfortunately passed on sending some of his therapists to the classes. The effectiveness was not lost, however, on the athletes Milton initially treated, and pro (and soon college) athletes began Bowen sessions, most in secret (during that time, athletes were barred from receiving any alternative healing).

People were flying in from all over the country for treatments, and because Milton grasped Bowen therapy so completely, they either wanted to take the seminar, or recommended a colleague. In every situation, he communicated his thorough understanding, and clients from several American cities pleaded with him to teach a class in their area. So with Ossie's willing approval, he also taught beginning classes throughout the country. Traveling to meet me in Queensland, Australia, in 1995, Milton assisted Ossie in classes and demonstrations on the Sunshine Coast, and taught one on his own in Eagle Heights, the town where my family lived.

1997 was eight years after he had first learned Bowen, and Milton thoroughly understood each of the 12 beginning lessons. In addition, he had developed a great many new moves, all based on Bowen. We named Milton's proposal Bowen Therapy International. The goals were to develop and promote Milton's interpretation of Tom Bowen's theories, plus establish and enforce instruction and quality control of these theories. Another goal of BTI was to promote research, in particular, Dr. JoAnne Whitaker's innovative studies (Dr. Whitaker had also been unceremoniously dropped).

Naturally, Milton's students and family (were shocked that he was being treated with such disrespect,) and they implored him to develop an advanced class quickly, so as to first introduce his more accomplished and comprehensive version. For this reason, Milton's premier class was an advanced level (Level IV), containing 14 innovative lessons. He felt a good instructor was only effective when they continued doing Bowen on a daily basis, and Milton enlisted advanced students who could instruct his work in other parts of the country. In addition, we traveled to Australia, where we researched Tom Bowen (and visited students and family). Milton's skillful mastery of Bowen therapy, as well as his quick wit, attracted people from many differing professions, and made his classes highly sought-after. We heard from pupils of all ages, that Bowen therapy classes with Milton Albrecht were truly mountaintop experiences... for both students and instructor.

The first Level I-II (beginning) class for Bowen Therapy International was held in June, 1999. Because Milton's practice was booked up about three weeks in advance (and because he was a perfectionist), writing the manual had been gradual. Using beautiful computer graphics, Milt enlisted a close friend, Doug Musso, (a dentist) to help him describe human anatomy. One page of the manual was devoted entirely to an explanation of Tom Bowen's philosophy (something that had not been done before). Milton also sprinkled his own theories throughout the lessons, always careful to define which thoughts were his own. He did not change Bowen's basic 12 beginning lessons, but developed easier, more accurate ways they could be learned and used. Neither Milton nor Tom Bowen had time to write down actual moves, and it was Milton's belief that Bowen often used differing procedures for similar ailments, depending on the client. He also felt that Bowen passed on very little of what he actually used, to the six men he taught. Because they all had different professions, each had interpreted Bowen's philosophies according to their own background.

Now through BTI, Milton continued to introduce Bowen to numerous health organizations, and was interviewed on local radio several times. In October, 1997, Milton and Dr. Whitaker traveled to San Diego for a presentation to the Academy of Environmental Medicine, the first traditional medical journal to recognize and publish empirical research on Bowen therapy. Milton's demonstration was such a hit, the next presenter was moved forward, and Milton was inundated by interested physicians. Several months later, my sister, Lois Larimore, had created and produced a TV show about alternative healing methods, and flew Milton to Toronto in November, 1999, for an interview. The show is called, "the Age of e", and the East Meets West episode can still be viewed throughout the world.

Certainly Milton enjoyed teaching and engaging in powerful discussion with an inquisitive public, but his first love was always the one-on-one experience with his clients. There were very few cases he couldn't help, and most were healed within one session. He would always ask family members to watch while he worked, explaining how they could help themselves in the future. Milton had bridged the gap between traditional and alternative medicine, and hospitals asked him to consult, and local medical doctors referred to him. In between clients, he could be found on the phone, describing a simple procedure the caller could use, nearly always with positive results.

Many times, Milton told me he believed he was "born to do Bowen", and awoke each morning excited about what new ailments and maladies would come through the door. Milton understood the body is its own best physician, and although the therapist's intent plays a role, it is important to not let the ego get in the way. Considering Milton's bodywork virtuosity, his humility was astonishing, his confidence supreme, yet subtle. He often remarked that the therapist should remember to get out of the way, "so nerves and muscles could remember their job descriptions".

Unfortunately, Milton's body sometimes had a difficult time remembering its own job description, and by 2000, was beginning to grow weary. Poor diet, stress and nicotine had gradually taken their toll, and even though he had quit drinking in the early 1990s, the combination was taking its toll on a cardiac system that was weak to begin with. (Although it's been written otherwise, Milton never drank while working on clients or teaching classes.) One of Milton's cardiac moves had improved heart rhythms, and because he experimented on himself whenever possible, had discovered its remarkable effects on his own intermittent heart murmur. But the worn down system had difficulty eliminating fluid, and he developed chronic obstructive pulmonary disease by 2002. On January 14, 2003, Milton made his passage to the next life, and although the cause of death was technically COPD, Milton's heart, and time, just gave out.

However, his heart goes on through every person who gives and receives Bowen Therapy in North America. Because of Milton's energetic, passionate promotion, Bowen Therapy continues on this continent today.

Sharing those years with Milt was a whirlwind experience, and I'm still here, long past my original prognosis, because I have continued to receive Bowen Therapy from 1989 to the present. Tom Bowen and Milton Albrecht were both extraordinary men, and for me, it has been an honor to have played just a small role in helping to introduce such a miraculous healing modality as Bowen Therapy.

My introduction to Milton
"When the patient is ready to heal – the healer will appear"

One Friday afternoon about September 1994 a patient told me about her foot pain and it sounded like an atypical sciatic nerve problem that was just showing up in her foot. I mentioned this and asked if she'd had any lower back problems? She said, "Oh no, it's not my sciatic nerve. I've had that before. This is different. I got that fixed two years ago." I inquired as to how she, "Got it fixed?" She told me that she'd had Bowen Therapy. I said, "I've never heard of that therapy. What's it about?" She replied, "It's kind of new here and most people don't know about it. The man who does it learned from the Australian people about two years ago, so that's why most people haven't heard of it." She told me about a practitioner in Auburn, California who'd been trained to do the treatments by the "Australian People." I asked if he was a chiropractor. She informed me that he was a Massage Therapist, but that he didn't do massage, only this Bowen technique.

I volunteered to her that I was suffering from lower back pain and sciatic nerve problems. She said, "Oh, you must go and see my friend. Not only has he helped me, but I've referred my boss, and my sister, and two of my neighbors, and he's helped us all with our back pains." I asked how to spell the gentleman's name so I could get his number from the phone-book to make an appointment. She said, "Oh no, you won't find him in the phone-book. He's got an unlisted number. I've got his card out in my car in the glove compartment, I'll go get it for you." After I finished my business with her foot she went out to her car and got the card. My receptionist copied it and gave me the copy and gave the patient back her card. Then she said, "Oh yeah. By the way, you must call him Monday through Friday from 8:00 AM to 9:00 AM. That's the only time of the day he answers the phone to make and change appointments, and if you call any other time and leave a message on his answering machine, he doesn't return calls." I thought, "That's a little odd?"

So, on Monday morning, I saw the note on my desk and glanced at the clock. It was 8:10 and I thought, "Good. I'm within the window of opportunity", so I dialed the number. It was busy, so, a few minutes later I tried again. Still busy, so I handed the task over to my receptionist with instructions to get me an appointment as soon as possible. About 5 minutes past 9:00 my receptionist informed me that he had a cancellation that afternoon at 5:00 which I could have; otherwise, the next available time was three weeks out. Not wanting to wait that long, I took the cancellation. That was the 3rd clue something was up; unlisted phone number, doesn't return calls, booked up three weeks out. When I arrived in his driveway that afternoon, there was an elderly lady sitting in one of those plastic $9.99 lawn chairs, missing a front tooth, and smoking a Camel cigarette. She said with a slight lisp, "If you're here to see Milton, you ring the bell he answers it himself." I thought to myself, "She's quite a receptionist, but I guess he doesn't let her do the phones?" The front door was open, while the screen door was shut. About a minute after ringing the chime, a man shuffled to the door to greet me. He was bare footed, wearing a pair of khaki shorts and a Hawaiian shirt, which was unbuttoned to the breastbone. He had a pack of cigarettes in his shirt pocket. He'd not shaved yet that day, and his hair was all mussed up. He said, "Are you Dr. Mosher?" I replied, "Yes, I am." He said, "How do you do? I'm Milton Albrecht. Come on in." As he led me through his house to a back bedroom I spotted a couple of biker-looking guys on the patio outside the kitchen working their way through a 12 pack of beer. The room was adorned with a map of Australia, a couple of boomerangs on the wall, an ammo belt on the chair, and a rifle standing in the corner. Now I'm thinking, "What did I just get myself into?" He asked me where I was hurting. I told him that my lower back on the right side around the lumbar-sacral area was the problem. He said, "Cool. I'll fix ya. Just lay on the table with your feet on the pillow, your butt in the air, and your face down in the cradle." I apprehensively complied.

During the treatment, many thoughts were racing through my mind. What was I doing here? How was a simple plucking of my muscles here and there going to relieve my back pain? Why'd he pluck a couple of muscles and leave the room for 3 to 5 minutes? Oh well, Ann my patient had relief, as well as all of the others she'd referred to this mystical man. After 10 to 15 minutes very deep relaxation set in and I almost fell asleep. One time he put his hand close to my low back and I could feel lots of heat radiating from me. He commented, "Ah Ha. You're cookin now!" After he turned me over onto my back, he moved the Adductor Magus muscle in my inner thigh and I thought I was going to hit the ceiling it hurt so much. I asked him if this was Rolfing, and he assured me that it wasn't. After he left the room for me to rest following the procedure, my palms started to sweat. It wasn't the usual watery kind of sweat, but a sticky - syrupy kind of discharge.

When he came back in the room and saw that I was patting my palms together, he touched my hand with his fingers and commented, "Ah Ha. That's toxins working their way out." I said, "Oh yeah. What kind of toxins?" a little facetiously. He sniffed his fingers and said, "Probably lactic acid cause it don't smell." I left it at that. Then he had me open my jaw and close it and said, "Your TMJ'S out." I recalled that I'd been nipping the inner side of my right cheek when chewing food the past few weeks. He had me make a knuckle with my index finger and place it between my teeth. He then tweaked a number of muscles around the jaw and temple area. Upon opening my jaw afterward, I could sense that my jaw was completely realigned. He instructed me to sit up. Upon arising from the table, I was a little light - headed.

Standing up after my head cleared, I couldn't believe how good I felt. I sensed more energy; the muscles all over my body were loose. My back didn't ache. Wow! the patient was right about this therapy. She'd referred her boss, sister and three friends to the therapist and he'd helped all of them, and now, me too. I commented that while he did nothing major to my back, but the pain was gone. He said, "There's nothing wrong with your back. Your *Adductor Magnus* was all locked up." I said, "What's that got to do with my back?" He said, "Everything. When that *Adductor* tightens the *Iliotibial band*, *Tensor Fascia Lata*, and *Gluteus Medius* muscles all tighten on the outer side of the hip in order to compensate. When you lift something and twist those tissues get strained, and then your back muscles go into spasm." I said, "That's exactly what's been happening. Whatever made that *Adductor* muscle lock up?" He said, "Dunnow-you must have built up lactic acid in them some time ago." I was so amazed at how good I felt and was so relieved to be rid of the pain, I didn't figure out the lactic acid issue till a few days later.

I asked how much I owed him for the treatment. He said, "Oh, just give me twenty bucks." As I handed him a $20 dollar bill, I asked, "How much do you usually charge? I'll be sending you some clients, as I grabbed a hand full of his business cards." He told me that his usual charge was $35.00, but he gave seniors a discount and kids were free. I asked if he was always booked three weeks out, and he said, "Yeah, except in the flu season and during the bad weather when the older folks don't like to drive, it slows down a little." Then I sprung the main question that was on my mind, "How many people do you treat every day?" He replied, "25 or 30!" I thought, "That's pretty good considering that he had very little overhead expenses."

While walking out to my car on my way to go home, I noticed that I was walking differently than before the treatment and the orthotics in my shoes were pressing up into my arch. So, I removed them and walked better without any arch support.

The night of the treatment I had such a good night's sleep I didn't move my head on the pillow at all. In the morning when I got out of bed my back wasn't stiff, the feet, legs and groin didn't ache, and I felt like a new person. I recalled that I didn't have jumpy-restless legs awaken me shortly after falling to sleep, and I didn't wake up with cramps in my calf muscles at 2:00 to 3:00 AM as I usually did.

A week later as I was dressing one morning, I saw that the hammertoes on my left foot had vanished. Sometime between the morning of discovery and the day of the treatment! I had to do a second take in order to believe my eyes. I did surgical procedures to straighten hammertoes and sometimes they didn't stay straight following surgery. Traditional stretching and physical therapy rarely helped them so I realized that this might be the missing piece to the puzzle. I couldn't wait to get to the telephone and call Milton in order to tell him about these miracles, plus to find out how I might learn how to perform some of the techniques.

After I told him all about what had happened since his treatment, he laughed and said, "That happens all the time". I jokingly told him, "I won't turn you in for practicing podiatry without a license if you'll show me how to do this for my patients." He asked me for my fax number so he could send me a brochure on a Bowen workshop he was teaching in January 1995, so I could sign up for it.

My first class with Milton

I attended a four-day workshop in Auburn California to learn the Bowen Technique in January 1995. At the beginning of the class Milt said, "I'm not no teacher, but I'm going to show you all how to do this Bowen stuff. I know that it might change some of your lives." I got a little pang in the pit of my solar plexus as he said that! The class covered Ossie's, 14 pages called "The Notes", which consisted of 23 different Bowen procedures including many foot and leg issues which were right up my alley. The notes were on colored construction paper and quite confusing to follow. Milt said this was so someone couldn't take a copy of them and learn how to do Bowen. They also covered many other procedures that were not within my scope of podiatry practice. I figured that I would sort it all out and find a way to use it all.

Eventually, I obtained a massage license so that I could legally touch a patient outside of my podiatry boundaries.

Working Bowen Therapy into my practice

Arriving at my office on Monday morning after the Bowen Class, the very first patient needed a Bowen treatment. She'd had a sciatic nerve problem in the past and she was certain that it had reoccurred because she had been performing floor exercises for long periods of time and now her left foot had a tingling sensation like the previous bout with sciatica.

After informing her about the new therapy I'd just learned, it took less than a nanosecond for her to ask if she could have a treatment that morning. She was escorted her into the operating room which I had transformed into a temporary therapy room and placed her on the surgical gurney which would serve as a massage table until one could be purchased. After checking my class notes I began the treatment. I only performed the treatment in the waist, legs, and feet to stay within the boundaries of my Podiatry license. When the session ended, she got up and stood on her feet she said, "It sure feels better. Not all the way, but at least by 50%."

The next morning, she called me to report, "That by noon Monday all of the symptoms had disappeared. The next time she got the sciatica back she would call me for treatment." I said, "To be sure she had a foot problem. And, thank you."

I eagerly began incorporating it into the podiatry practice. The first week I treated 12 patients with it. Six of them returned the following week for a second session. One of them said, "Dr. Mosher, I don't know what you did? But, you've changed my life!" Then, he explained how. Another said, "Dr. Mosher, you won't believe what happened after that treatment you did last week!" Then, she told me what happened. One other said, "I had a runner's high all day after the treatment. And, now I feel a sense of wellbeing and balance." Another one said, "If only the medical doctors would take this holistic and natural approach to our health care issues."

As the months passed by, many would say, the same things or, "I sure wish that I had met you sooner so that my life could've been better. I've been through years of hell."

Thousands of patients experienced similar results from the treatments that I did and <u>all were from what Milt taught me!</u>

Chats with Milton during and after my Bowen sessions

Arrhythmia:

One of my favorite stories, which pretty much sums up Milton, was the one about an elderly lady client of his who was having problems with a cardiac arrhythmia. After a couple of sessions she discontinued her heart medication, and seemed to do just fine. When she went to her cardiologist at the University Medical Center for her follow-up appointment, she informed him of what she had done. He immediately performed an EKG, which was quite normal, and could not believe his eyes. He compared the present strip with the last one, and asked her more about what she had done. She told the cardiologist about her Bowen sessions and gave him Milton's name and phone number. Also she gave him specific instructions to call Milton on Monday through Friday between 8:00 and 9:00 AM. He called Milton the next morning to learn more about Bowen, and asked if Milton could possibly come to the Medical Center and show and tell about the process. Milton replied, 'Hell no", and, hung up on him!

Optional Procedure:

Milton first taught me this procedure during one of our fireside chats circa 2000. Initially he taught it in his Basic Bowen course. However, he discovered that the students only practiced the one procedure because it worked so well, and they neglected the rest of the Basic lessons. So, he moved it to the "Advanced" section of his training.

He told me to, "Use this when your client is in so much pain that they can't get up on the table. It will relax them so they can move a little better, and then they can get up on the table." I filed this into my data bank and went about my business. On occasion, I found this procedure helpful for patients who were in acute spasms and could not climb up onto the table. It enabled them to be slightly more mobile, and it only took a minute or so to do.

K.C, who was one of my long-time, regular podiatry patients said, "Oh my gosh. I met your guru, Uncle Milty. I went to his house with a friend and he cleared up my gallbladder problem. Just to think that I was going to have surgery for my gallbladder. Now I won't need it!" I was happy for her and we talked a bit about Milton and Bowen during the rest of her podiatry visit that morning.

After Milton passed in January of 2003, K.C. was in for her podiatry appointment. She lamented, "Oh, I sure wish our Uncle Milty was still here. My gallbladder problem has resurfaced and my doctor wants me to have surgery. I'm getting a second opinion tomorrow. I remember how he fixed my problem and that was over 4 years ago." I said, "I can give you a Bowen session." She said, "Oh! That's right. I forgot you do Bowen too. I'll schedule an appointment after I get my second opinion." I overheard my nurse bringing K.C. into one of my Bowen rooms. She said, "This is your first Bowen with Dr. Mosher isn't it? You need to take your shoes off and lay face down on the table with your feet on the pillow and your face in the face cradle." K.C. replied, "Oh no. I don't have to lie down for this. We can just do it standing up." I was on to what she was referring to so, I quickly stepped in to save an argument. I said, "K.C. you mean to tell me that all Milton did for you that time you saw him was the standing-up procedure?" She replied, "That's right. He did it right there in his living room and I was fine all those years." So, I did the standing Optional Procedure for her. I talk to my former office staff now and then, and they keep me posted on patients I was fond of, and she has been fine ever since.

At massage school I performed this procedure on a number of classmates who had gallbladder problems with equally good results.

<u>Waits and number of procedures during a session:</u>

As the years went by Milton started doing more of the procedure parts during a segment of the session and extending the waits rather than how I originally learned from his assistants and he - as is shown in the Full Sequence in the Files section on the Facebook group – Bowen Therapy Worldwide. He figured that the body could respond to the larger clusters of moves as long as the rest period was long enough to do so. How he knew how long was long enough, I do not know. Milt seemed to develop more medical intuitive skills during the latter part of his life.

Other Milton stories of interest

<u>Shoulder Procedure:</u>

One Sunday afternoon, I stopped by one of Milton's Bowen classes to say hi, and see what was doing. He was in the middle of demonstrating the "Frozen Shoulder Procedure". After the demonstration he told a story about a friend of his who one Sunday morning called to see if he could do a session to relieve his friend's frozen shoulder.

Milt said, "Leave me alone. This is my day off. Call me in the morning", and hung up. About an hour later the doorbell rang and here was his buddy standing there, holding his arm up to un-weight the shoulder. He said, "Come on Milt. Please give me a treatment. I can't move my shoulder". Milt said, "Come on in, but damn it and I told you I am not working today. Which shoulder hurts?" His friend indicated which one, and Milt had him turn to the opposite side. Milt hit him as hard as he could with his fist on the non-painful shoulder. The friend cried, "What did you do?" Milt said, "I just fixed your shoulder-shut up." His friend said, "No. You made my good shoulder hurt." Milt said, "Try out the bad one." When he did, the pain and stiffness was all gone. Is this an "Advanced Procedure?" I promptly went home and tried it on my wife who had been experiencing off and on shoulder pain for the past 6 months. We had done all the Bowen procedures. She had been to physical therapy. NSAIDS were about her only relief. After the ringing of the bell (striking her good shoulder), she experienced an intense healing crisis in the affected shoulder, after which, she has never had another pain.

Carpal Tunnel:
Since Milt knew everyone in town and was a very popular figure, he attended lots of parties, weddings, and festivities. When someone had a carpal tunnel problem in the *right wrist*, Milt would do the arm procedure on the *left arm*. Low and behold the carpal tunnel would disappear. Sometimes this resulted in cancelled surgeries and MRI appointments. Milt knew that the body-mind - nervous system doesn't know the right from the left. This is the same as when his buddy had relief of shoulder pain on one side when the pain was evoked on the opposite shoulder.

Teeth and meridians:
The extraction of a bad tooth as recommended by Milt often cleared up his
client's symptoms. Multiple extractions led to dementia in some of his clients.

Ganglions:
At one of our fireside chats, he told me that ganglionic cysts were caused by an overload of caffeine. He told me that when he "popped" the cysts for his clients, many times they had sleepless nights following. I Thought, "Oh yeah. Sure". There was a large one behind my ankle when he told me this. At the time, I drank eight to ten cups of coffee a day. I cut down to two cups and about three months later, the cyst was 80% reduced in size. After three more months, it was gone! He was right-on once again.

The Ugly Sister Procedure:
Occasionally Milt would awaken in the morning and call his sister Debbie and tell her about a procedure that he had dreamed about the night before. He would try it out on her that morning and then he called it the Ugly Sister Procedure X.

At Milton's Memorial Service 2003:
A young lady who was a college student stood up and told about her Milton experience. Her mother was a client of Milton's. The daughter had a science class assignment in high school to write a paper about some type of health care therapy. She asked Milton if she could observe him work and ask some questions in order to write her paper. Of course Milt said yes. She spent a number of afternoons after school with Milt. She presented Milt with a copy of the paper when it was done. He was so taken by what she had written he enrolled her in one of his classes with her tuition waived. She was forever grateful to him for all of what his services were about and for teaching her how to do Bowen Therapy.

Milt's connection to Tom:
Milt often told me that he was aware of Tom's presence while he was working on clients and while he was working things out.

Stories from other students, friends, relatives, and clients:

Cousin Albert:
Hundreds of my patients have told me that during the rest periods while on the table they felt euphoric. Or, others felt a runner's high for a few hours after their session. A result of beta endorphin release from the node points.

Hundreds of patients came for sessions to help them sleep, relax during a test, reduce their stress level, and improve their overall sense of well-being.

Thousands of my patients fell asleep during their rest periods, which were sometimes 10 to 15 minutes long. Hundreds of my patients went on to healing of old wounds, injuries, and surgeries which were unfinished business.

Made in the USA
Columbia, SC
29 April 2025